The Complete
MASTER CLEANSE

The Complete
MASTER CLEANSE

A Step-by-Step Guide to
Maximizing the Benefits
of **The Lemonade Diet**

Tom Woloshyn

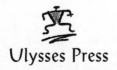

Ulysses Press

Published by: Ulysses Press
          P.O. Box 3440
          Berkeley, CA 94703
          www.ulyssespress.com

ISBN10: 1-56975-613-9
ISBN13: 978-1-56975-613-3
Library of Congress Control Number: 2006938936

Printed in the United States by Bang Printing

10 9 8 7 6 5 4 3

Acquisitions Editor: Nicholas Denton-Brown
Managing Editor: Claire Chun
Editor: Mark Woodworth
Editorial and production staff: Ruth Marcus, Lisa Kester, Tamara Kowalski,
    Lauren Harrison
Index: Sayre Van Young
Cover design: DiAnna Van Eycke
Cover photo: ©photos.com

Illustrations on page 120 courtesy of Dr. Bernard Jensen; photos on page 156 reproduced from image library of Division of Parasitic Diseases, Centers for Disease Control and Prevention; case study photos on page 166 courtesy of (*left*) BlessedHerbs.com and (*right*) Dr. Jensen; author portrait on page 200 by Frances Litman.

Distributed by Publishers Group West

NOTE TO READERS
This book has been written and published strictly for informational and educational purposes only. It is not intended to serve as medical advice or to be any form of medical treatment. You should always consult your physician before altering or changing any aspect of your medical treatment and/or undertaking a diet regimen, including the Master Cleanse diet as described in this book. Do not stop or change any prescription medications without the guidance and advice of your physician. Any use of the information in this book is made on the reader's good judgment after consulting with his or her physician and is the reader's sole responsibility. This book is not intended to diagnose or treat any medical condition and is not a substitute for a physician.

Contents

Acknowledgments

I would like to thank Stanley Burroughs for his consistent and unwavering commitment to his life's work. Although he faced much opposition and ridicule, he was undaunted by forces that at times made his life difficult. He created a sound, yet simple, system of healing that is available to almost anyone who takes the time and effort to experience it.

I also wish to thank my instructor, Maynard Dalderis, who dedicated himself to properly learning Stanley's work by taking his training multiple times. Maynard was an adept and proficient teacher who made Stanley's work so exciting and credible that it inspired me and many like me to take this knowledge and bring it to others.

Richard Grassie and Michael Liggett were also instrumental in getting me on my newfound life path, and for that I am extremely grateful to them.

To Shannon Buchan, my former wife, who never made me get a job when I found it difficult to make the rent for some months when I began my healing work. I also thank her for helping me write this book and giving me many suggestions to make it a better one. Her constant focus helped me keep my attention on the work at hand.

Thanks also to Tamara Olson for supporting me in my endeavors in finding adjuncts to the Master Cleanse and for always believing in my life's mission.

I would also like to express my gratitude to the many thousands of people who trusted me to support them during their health challenges, so that they might heal themselves. This body of experience that I gained from them has taught me much, which I can now share with others who are looking to enhance their health and seeking the empowerment that they deserve.

I cannot forget to thank both my editor, Mark Woodworth, for his patience and his wonderful editing skill, and the rest of the staff at Ulysses Press, including Nick Denton-Brown, for giving me an opportunity to fulfill my long-held desire by writing this book.

Finally, thank you to the Creative Power that makes all things possible.

PART 1

Origin of the Master Cleanse

CHAPTER 1

Why You Need This Book

For many years, clients and friends whom I have treated for various health problems have asked me to write a book such as this. They have benefited from my guidance, because of the extensive knowledge I have developed with the Master Cleanse and my experience in using it, as well as my relationship with its creator and developer (who will be profiled in Chapter 3) and one of his foremost students and teachers, Maynard Dalderis.

Recent articles about the efficacy of the Master Cleanse have been featured in leading American newspapers and on top-rated television shows, with a variety of celebrity endorsements, bringing it the attention it so rightly deserves.[1] The Master Cleanse is a marvelous gift to those tens or even hundreds of thousands of people who are looking for a simple, inexpensive, and amazingly effective way to improve their health, boost their sense of well-being (both physical and emotional), and change from their experience of *dis-ease* (as I will spell it throughout this book) to a steady state of feeling healthy and whole.

What Is the Master Cleanse?

The Master Cleanse is one of the most simple, effective, and inexpensive cleansing and healing programs available. It is a liquid monodiet (that is, one mixture only) designed to work with and complement your body's own cleansing and detoxifying processes, and at the same time to nourish your body with the things it needs to function. It is *not* a true fast (one in which there is no nutrition), nor is it a means to starve the body in order to lose weight dangerously fast. The cleanse is typically done for 10 days, but can be safely maintained for many more days in a row, even weeks, when desired.

The ingredients of the monodiet are specified in detail in Part 2 of this book, but for now you will be glad to know that they are readily available, light on the wallet, and easy to combine and drink: good water, fresh lemon juice, maple syrup, and cayenne pepper. That's all.

I have benefited greatly from this program! For more than two decades I have followed my own instructions for doing the Master Cleanse, correcting my steps as I learned from experience, tailoring the program to my clients with a variety of conditions, and on occasion testing and adding other therapies as adjuncts. I have completed over one hundred cleanses of my own body, and can bear personal witness to its health-giving benefits. I would not recommend it if it did not work for me. Among the most important benefits it has brought me:

- I have not seen a medical doctor for treatment from the first day I began training in this program, January 8, 1980.
- For over 25 years I have used this program to treat all of my own health conditions, including neck and shoulder pain, prostate issues, headaches, constipation, shingles, and other minor ailments.
- I have gained confidence and freedom by knowing that with the Master Cleanse I can deal with those health issues that arise for me.

Despite the thousands of successful Master Cleanse treatments I have helped clients do in my practice, and the hundreds of success stories I have heard from colleagues and other reputable sources, there are still many naysayers of the program. No surprise here! This is how a society typically reacts to virtually any holistic or "unconventional" nonmedical health practice throughout history, as well as to scientific discoveries that are later borne out by careful research.

Today, even though we are well launched into the 21st century and living in an age of supposed rationality, many people do not understand the simple concept of what causes, and cures, organic *dis-ease*. This is true partly because of the monopoly of the health care system by allopathic medicine, otherwise known as mainstream medicine. This monopoly makes every effort to discredit the alternative health care movement that has been carefully built on traditional folk-treatments dating back hundreds of years through myriad cultures.

GOOD TO KNOW

Dis-ease has its origins in the 14th century. The Middle English word *disese*, combining *des- + eise*, meant a condition of an animal, or one of its parts, that impairs normal functioning and is often manifested by outward signs or inner symptoms. The root *ease* derives from the Old French and Latin for *adiacens*, or "lying down." *Dis-ease* implies the inability to rest comfortably and feel well.

Doubters and Skeptics

When I started practicing in my field of holistic health counseling, about a quarter century ago, the medical establishment held fast to the pervasive ideology that diet had little or no effect in causing dis-ease. Doctors treated patients as if their bodies had no necks to connect the mind and body, as one being. Their patients' diet and state of mind were believed to be of little or no consequence to their bodies' health. It was thought that people could eat whatever they desired, live however they wished, and if they developed symptoms of a dis-ease their doctor could prescribe a magic pill or potion, or do a little operation, that would "fix" all their problems, which seemed to be of unknown origin.

In recent years, however, more and more of us in the holistic health field have learned that mind and body *are* connected and, therefore, that any dis-ease or illness must be treated in a unified and complementary manner that takes both into account.

To give only one example, in February 2007 a medical study in Canada found that the children of women who took a prenatal multivitamin while pregnant went on to have significantly lower incidences of certain cancers.[2] Brain tumors were reduced by 27 percent, leukemia by 39 percent, and neuroblastoma (an often fatal dis-ease of embryonic ganglion cells) by 47 percent. It would have been heresy, 25 years ago, to suggest that expectant mothers could, with a simple supplement, have such a dramatic impact on their children's health in the months or years to come.

Some researchers have even reported that grants to study diet as a potential cause of cancer were in the past almost always turned down by funders who favor mainstream medicine, or who are financially linked to it in some way.

Over the years, as I developed my holistic practice, many people have scoffed, even laughed in my face, telling me that I was crazy to suggest a link between dis-ease and diet...that no scientific evidence would support this...that my explanation was too simplistic...that the Master Cleanse had no basis in medical science...and on and on. In my view, such people simply did not want to hear the bad news: that they literally were making themselves sick by their own lifestyle choices. And they didn't want to hear the good news, either: that I could help them feel better with my program.

The Key to Success: Doing the Cleanse Correctly

I know the Master Cleanse works, when done correctly. I have talked to thousands of people about the Master Cleanse. I have often been astonished to realize that a large percentage of those who have done the Master Cleanse have done it wrong. Some people use poor or inappropriate ingredients, or in the wrong proportions, or add an idea of their own, or come off the cleanse too early, or sneak food when they feel hunger pangs during the cleanse. That is why I have written this book—to present an easy-to-follow, complete program of cleansing, as well as supplemental information on adjuncts to cleansing.

Recently I was in a health food store buying lemons. When the cashier said she was on a fast, I asked her which one. She said "the Lemonade Diet"—that is, the Master Cleanse itself—and she was on Day 3. I replied that, by coincidence, I too was on Day 3 just then. I then asked her a few questions. It quickly became clear to me that she was omitting one very important step, so I gently told her about it, and explained my practice a little to give her some confidence in what I was saying. (Of course, I was not treating her professionally.)

This happens almost every day with me, and sometimes several times a day when I'm circulating at conferences or teaching workshops. The sad truth is that a great many people seem unable (or unwilling?) to follow the directions to do the Master Cleanse correctly. This virtually ensures that they will not succeed, and can even cause many who do the cleanse improperly to experience much grief and later feel disdain for trying any kind of cleanse ever again.

Such unfortunate mistakes hinder the huge potential of the Master Cleanse to help those many people who are looking for answers to improve their health and well-being. Further, such mistakes make an already misunderstood concept of natural health seem even more suspect in many seekers' minds.

How This Book Is Structured

This book has been carefully designed to instruct you how to do the Master Cleanse in the most effective way possible, to achieve the greatest benefits to your health and well-being. The chapters in **Part I** will provide you the intriguing background of the visionary man who developed the Master Cleanse, tell you why today most of us need to cleanse our bodies regularly, help you understand the physical and emotional aspects of dis-ease, and explain how the cleanse works to detoxify the body.

Part II lists step-by-step procedures for getting ready to do the cleanse, gathering the necessary ingredients and learning their properties, doing the cleanse correctly and safely, staying on it for the right duration for optimal results, coming off it feeling well, and dealing with any issues or concerns that might arise along the way. A day-by-day chart is presented, giving you a place to log your intake and to note how you feel each day; it will provide a helpful record for future cleanses as well.

Part III contains chapters explaining several adjunctive therapies that can support the Master Cleanse. It also features chapters that increase your understanding of how the mind can help the body get better, explain how you can rid yourself of harmful parasites that treat your body as a host to feed on, and offer other useful information such as advanced cleansing techniques.

Finally, the book contains a variety of *answers* to frequently asked questions, inspiring *testimonials* from people who now swear by the Master Cleanse, some of my favorite *recipes* for healthful eating after doing a cleanse, and lastly some *resources* and *further reading* to help you in your quest for better health.

I devoutly hope that this book will inspire you—and perhaps some of your friends or family as well—to take your health safely back into your own hands. Doing a Master Cleanse can be one of the most empowering and satisfying things you could ever do for yourself! The rewards you experience from it will go far beyond what you might ever have expected or thought you deserved. And, believe me, I am confident that you will want to continue to do Master Cleanses regularly, for the rest of your happy and healthy life. I strongly support you in achieving your goals.

So now plunge in, read on, and enjoy this book. *Your life may never be the same again!*

CHAPTER 2

How I Found the Master Cleanse

In my young adulthood I had taken a mindless job: working as the driver of a front-end loader moving steel around at a mill. My part-time job had became full time, and for a while I had put going back to school low on my list of priorities. My work afforded me the time to let my mind wander. One day I found myself saying, "I want to be healthier, I want to be happier, and I want to be more fulfilled." I would then repeat this frequently, like a mantra. One day everything changed. But first I have to tell you how the pieces came together.

Diving Into My New Life

I had always had a desire to skydive—that's right, jumping out of airplanes. OK, so call me crazy, call me a risk taker, but you know the adage: "Nothing ventured, nothing gained." The desire to skydive led me to an instructor in the sport who later became a friend, named Michael Liggett. In his early years of skydiving Michael had spent time in California, where he met a woman who introduced him to an alternative lifestyle in which he chose to eat more consciously and to start taking nutritional supplements. After a couple of years of friendship, Michael moved in with my partner and me. While we were roommates he was dating a woman who gave him a book called *Healing for the Age of Enlightenment*, by someone named Stanley Burroughs. She had received the book from a former boyfriend, named Richard Grassie, who had just returned from Hawaii, where he happened to meet Burroughs and became intrigued with his work. Well, Michael's girlfriend passed the book on to him, he read it, and he talked to me about a so-called "Lemonade Diet," or the "Master Cleanser®," that the book claimed could heal your every ailment.

Being very skeptical I replied, "If it's so good, why don't doctors use it?" (One of those questions that has no answer.) I said that I wasn't interested, but Michael persisted. I told him that I had reservations about doing the diet because of my work at the steel mill. I felt that it might be dangerous, because, as I said, "What if I got weak and fainted?"

In those days I was eating meat twice or three times a day and drinking a quart of milk daily; at the time, I thought mine was a healthy diet. I believed my health to be good, so I certainly didn't need a weird "lemonade diet." Truth be known, I had a bowel movement only every two to three days, which was called normal by medical standards. I was also experiencing a lot of pain in my neck and shoulders from injuries to my neck while playing football and from a compression injury I sustained at work.

Around that time my doctor suggested that I have some vertebrae in my neck fused, to stop the pain—a radical treatment. I was actually considering this as an option. This sounds crazy in retrospect, I realize, but we all do the best we can with what we know at the time.

As fate would have it, the workers at my plant went out on strike. Now I had the time to do the Lemonade Diet while off work. So I told Michael that I would do it, mainly to prove to him that it wouldn't work! Then all three of us—Michael, my girlfriend, and I—decided to try the lemonade drill. On the third day of the diet, I went to my dentist to get my wisdom teeth removed, one per week for four weeks. After doing some surgery and removing the first tooth, the dentist gave me two prescriptions to take, an antibiotic and a painkiller. I told him that I was on a diet that recommended not taking drugs while doing it, and actually defended this position. He pressed me and said that an infection could spread from the gum to the heart and kill me. I knew someone who had died in this manner, so I acknowledged that this was a valid point.

I then went on the antibiotics and stopped the Lemonade Diet for a while, perhaps for 4 to 6 days. Then I went back on it and continued to have my dental work done, but refused to take the drugs. Each socket healed so quickly that I would remove the stitches myself and never experienced any pain whatsoever. Not only did my gums heal quickly, but after doing the Master Cleanse I started having a bowel movement every day like clockwork, an important improvement in my health.

When I started eating again after coming off the diet properly, I came to two realizations. First, after eating a small rib-eye steak one evening, I felt as if I had consumed a lead brick; how could I possibly digest that? Second, drinking a glass of milk the next day also made me feel uncomfortable. Hey, what was happening to me? My two favorite foods made me feel heavy, as if my insides were ill at ease.

Years after this experience, as I began building my holistic health practice, I would recommend the Master Cleanse to many people who were having tooth or gum problems. One client who came to me mostly for weight loss was on the Master Cleanse and, on her 28th day of the diet, went in for a root canal. When the dentist removed the cap, she was so surprised at what she saw that she called in a second dentist to view the tooth; the infection in the root was now completely gone—something they had never seen occur before. My client, of course, was happy to forgo the root canal and save herself the extra expense and pain.

We Become How We Were Raised

As children, we usually were not given choices about the food we ate. We were told to clean our plate, otherwise we wouldn't get dessert, or we should eat every last bit because children in Africa were starving. We learned to numb our feelings, even our bodies, to cope, and so we adopted our parents' way of eating as our own lifestyle. I have since learned that the Master Cleanse will resensitize your body to whatever you put into it. After some experimentation with the diet, I was now experiencing and enjoying many foods in a completely different way.

There I was, a confirmed carnivore, now apparently unable to eat meat or drink milk in comfort. People would ask me what was wrong. I would reply that I just felt better if I didn't eat those things, and again they asked what was up with that. Eventually I would have to tell them, "You can eat what *you* want, and I will choose to eat what feels good to me, thank you very much."

Some of my clientele, when they are preparing to do the Master Cleanse, have said to me, "Tom, I am not here to become a vegetarian," and I have responded that I had no intention of making them one, nor could I even if I wanted to. A month later these people would tell me that they had eaten meat only once that month and didn't miss it at all.

I believe that everyone makes their best choices when they have been given enough information to understand all their options, as well as the consequences of those choices.

My First Master Cleanse

In spring 1979 I had my first cleanse. A short time later, while wrestling with my brother, I suffered an injury to my urethra, which got an infection that spread to my prostate gland. This event caused me much pain and embarrassment for several months. I started taking a number of prescription drugs, none of which worked. The first drug caused an allergic reaction that left

90 percent of my body covered with an intensely itchy rash. My experience with two urologists was nothing short of horrific. You might be asking yourself why, instead, I didn't use the Master Cleanse again. I guess I thought a bacteria or a fungus had invaded my body and had to be killed, hence my trusting visits to the doctors. I told myself that medical professionals knew how to take care of such things,

As fate would have it, Richard Grassie, the man who had met Stanley Burroughs in Hawaii, brought a man named Maynard Dalderis to the city where I lived, to teach a workshop on Burroughs's work. This workshop taught not only the use of the Master Cleanse but also his other important works, Vita-Flex and Color Therapy (see Chapters 7 and 8 for full descriptions of these adjunctive therapies).

I attended the introductory lecture and was so impressed that I decided to attend the workshop itself, which started the next day. On the first day we heard a lecture on the Master Cleanse, and consequently all but two of us students went on the cleanse in the next day or so. After about four days my instructor, Maynard, asked me, in front of the entire class, why I wasn't on the cleanse. I replied that I had already done it once. He suggested that I go on it again and I told him that I was resistant and of course he asked why again. I said I didn't like the taste of the lemonade, so he asked me how I made it. I explained that I had done the Master Cleanse with commercial lemons, a commonly found light maple syrup, cayenne, and water. After drinking lemonade for a few days, I said, I couldn't stand the taste anymore, so I would take two tablespoons of lemon juice, and then take two tablespoons of maple syrup, followed by two capsules of cayenne pepper and then a glass of water. By now everyone in the workshop was laughing uproariously. Maynard suggested that I get organic lemons, buy a dark grade of maple syrup, and put the cayenne, in powder form, into the drink each time I made it. He assured me that I would find it much more palatable if I made it correctly. Follow the instructions, was the message I heard.

Using the Correct Method

The next time I went on the Master Cleanse, having been wised up and now being in possession of a great deal more information, things went well. I enjoyed the drink, and to my surprise by Day 4 my prostate infection was no longer a problem. If you have never had a prostate infection, let me explain some of the symptoms: difficult urination, painful urination, and pain at the end of the penis (where the nerve endings of the prostate gland surface). You can imagine my relief when, as if by a miracle, these symptoms, which I had been experiencing for several months, disappeared completely.

I continued on the cleanse for 16 days and then stopped. I took the next 3 days to come off the diet, went back to eating for 3 days, and then went back on the cleanse for another 12 days. I came off it once more and ate for 3 more days, and then went back on the cleanse for 10 more days. This meant doing the cleanse for 38 out of 50 days. I continued doing the cleanse through 1980 on and off, until I had done 100 days in total. I had been truly Master Cleansed, to the nth degree!

At that point I felt as good as I have ever felt in my life. I had lost about nine pounds by the end and was quite thin, which concerned some people. Caring friends and even acquaintances would ask which cult I belonged to and how much money did I send to them (that being a time when cults were popular).

My Current Master Cleanse Schedule

These days, having a good deal of experience with the Master Cleanse of varying durations, I like to do a maintenance program. It consists of at least four, 10-day cleanses per year. Actually, at the time of composing this section of the book I am on Day 6 of a cleanse, and yet I'm writing with a clear head and a steady hand. I have now probably done more than 1,000 days of the Master Cleanse over the years.

You might ask, "Why so much?" The answer is obvious. Think of it as an exercise program. Would you work out for one week, or one month, or one year and then stop, never to repeat your workout and thinking that you had reached the pinnacle of physical perfection? No, if you were smart you would continue to exercise to keep fit—so, with the same thinking, you should cleanse your body regularly, as part of an ongoing healthy lifestyle.

It's critical that you understand that your first step is to get yourself well enough to go on and live a healthier life. The second step is to do the maintenance work to keep up what you have created, and build on the results. Depending on your state of overall health, this can take 50, 100, or more days of cleansing in a one-year period to get yourself as healthy as you can get by doing the Master Cleanse.

For myself, after the first 100 days of cleansing I began to feel as good while eating a healthy diet as I had when on the Master Cleanse. Through experience I have found that most people only feel their best while on the Master Cleanse, and it is not until they've done several cleanses that they feel just as good while eating food as when they are cleansing.

But back to my story. I was soon to meet the Master Cleanser himself...

CHAPTER 3

My Story with Stanley

In 1986 I went to visit Stanley Burroughs in California. I had talked to Stanley over several years on the phone, asking him questions and ordering books, and we had become friends, but this was to be my first face-to-face meeting. Stanley picked me up at the Sacramento airport. He was then 82. While driving me to his home he told me about his experience of taking a driver's test. As part of the test they did an eye exam, and told him that he needed to wear glasses while driving. So he purchased new eyeglasses but found them annoying to wear. If you have read Stanley's work, you know he has written up a recipe for eyedrops. He went on to say that he made up a bottle of his eyedrops and proceeded to use them for a time. He said it gave him great joy when he went back to the Department of Motor Vehicles a year later to redo his eye exam, only to learn that he no longer needed to wear glasses at all.

Shortly after we arrived at Stanley's home, he asked me to give him a Vita-Flex treatment, involving pressure-point massage. (This adjunctive therapy is described in detail in Chapter 7.) Over the course of the session he was so astounded by my ability to do Vita-Flex that he asked me at least three times who had taught me, and I kept replying, "Maynard."

Maynard Dalderis was my teacher. He had taken Stanley's training 10 times, because Stanley, even though gifted in many areas, was not the best teacher. With his hard work and commitment, Maynard made an intense effort to learn Stanley's work. I was fortunate to have had Maynard teaching me, because he was by far the best teacher of Stanley's work at the time. Stanley did teach me some vital things about his work, but most of all he spoke to me of his many experiences in the field of health and told me some of his personal history.

The Body's Auras

Stanley started his lifetime of healing work by attending training in 1925 or 1926 given by a Colonel Dinshah Ghadiali in the use of Color Therapy. Since childhood, Stanley had been able to see auras, or the body's bioelectromagnetic field. It was a gift little understood during most of his life. These fields, or auras, can now be measured by scientific equipment. He quickly could see that shining a light of a certain color on a person's body could have a positive influence on that person's well-being and health. If this seems too weird, just think of it for a minute: If there were no light, would there be any life? (I will delve much deeper into Color Therapy in Chapter 8.)

In the late 1920s, Stanley Burroughs had been a vaudeville performer. A booking agent he knew had suffered a stroke and lay bedridden, paralyzed on one side. Stanley wanted to help, so he approached him about using the Color Therapy he had learned and offered to treat him, at no charge. Within one week the man was up and walking and had returned to his job. Of course, this apparent miracle won Stanley great credibility.

His next client was a woman who had contracted syphilis. In those days no antibiotics were available for that condition, and what paltry treatment was available lasted six months and cost some $200 (a fortune then). Stanley said he would treat her with Color Therapy and charge her only $25 if the treatment worked. Two weeks later she went for a second test, and found that her syphilis was now gone.

Stanley considered Color Therapy to be extremely effective for most conditions, though there was one condition that took a long time to heal: stomach ulcers. Stanley thought it was simply unacceptable that, even when treated with Color Therapy, ulcers took up to six months to heal.

A Bolt of Wisdom from Out of the Blue

He searched for solutions to the ulcer puzzle, but nothing came of it until 1941 when, while sitting down for dinner one evening, he was inspired to write. He quickly jotted down the instructions for a Lemonade Diet, which would win him fame. This sudden urge to write he later called "divine inspiration."

As fate would have it, one day later there came a knock at Stanley's door. There stood a gentleman who had just been to his doctor with a bleeding ulcer. The doctor had told him that he needed to have surgery almost immediately, or he would soon die. Stanley then handed him the piece of paper he had just written on the day before. The man looked at the paper and said with annoyance, "Lemon juice? Cayenne pepper? I can't eat those foods!"

Stanley asked him, "How long have you had your ulcer?"

"Three years," the man replied.

Stanley asked, "Have you ever eaten lemon or cayenne pepper in those three years?"

"No," he said.

Stanley again asked, "Did your ulcer get better or get worse in those three years?"

The answer, of course, was that it had become worse. Stanley thought for a moment and, with some logic, said, "You haven't eaten lemon or cayenne pepper in three years and your ulcer only got worse. Maybe cayenne pepper and lemon are the very foods you need to eat." With this the man said he would try this diet, but felt sure it would be a painful process. On Day 5 the man called on Stanley again, to report that he had not experienced any pain yet but expected to, any day now. Stanley assured him that his pain would not return and that he would be fine. On Day 11 he again appeared, this time with an X-ray showing that his ulcer had completely healed. Stanley felt convinced that he had discovered something that would help others.

The Master Cleanser® Is Named

As a result of this formative incident, for many years Stanley used what he termed the "Lemonade Diet" primarily to treat ulcers. Eventually, his clients reported that many other conditions cleared up or improved dramatically, beyond their ulcers healing. It became obvious to Stanley that the Lemonade Diet was a cleansing program that helped virtually any condition to improve and often heal. He renamed it the "Master Cleanser®." Eventually he wrote up his findings and recommendations. (See Chapter 6.)

Through the great many successes that thousands of people have experienced by using the Master Cleanse over the years, Stanley Burroughs's work has gained much attention. And I believe that now people are ready to embrace his other works as well, with the goal of attaining even more significant and welcome results in improved health and well-being.

But first we must explore why we need to cleanse our bodies at all. After all, doesn't nature do all the work for us? Don't our bodily systems keep purring along automatically, helping us to function at our best, if we just ingest a bit of any old food and drink now and then? Read on for the answer.

CHAPTER 4

Why Do We Need to Cleanse?

Many medical professionals would say that the body can cleanse itself just fine. It does not need extreme diets and programs and therapies to function well, they assert. But I could not disagree more strongly. Would you never bathe your body during your entire life? Would you never launder your clothes? Would you never clean your house? Would you never disinfect and sparkle up your bathroom?

Some of these medical professionals would poison you with an arsenal of drugs to fight the ever-increasing number of dis-eases that our culture, our environment, and our lifestyle throw at us. Doctors like these will cut deep into the body and throw away the diseased parts, or take parts from someone else and put them back into you, or implant manufactured devices in your body. When all these fail to work, doctors can always radiate you with high-energy beams to kill some dysfunctional part of your body, or prescribe the latest wonder drug, with all the wonderful side effects mentioned so blithely on TV commercials. You ask yourself, "Might such surgical, pharmaceutical, and therapeutic interventions have some extremely serious side effects?" "Well," you are told, "you just have to roll with the punches. After all, we're here to *help* you."

Looked at from this perspective, that sounds somewhat frightening. Is it possible that a cure can be more deadly than the dis-ease itself? Why, if you were in your right mind, would you willingly put yourself through such an ordeal?

You would do so when you are governed by fear. It is fear and ignorance that make people feel powerless in the health care system that dominates in America today. When frightened, people will logically look to authority figures and let them take control of their lives. Like sheep, people are herded into clinics or hospitals, blindly believing in those well-established and trusted institutions without ever questioning what they are putting themselves at risk to do, or how well a recommended procedure or drug might work.

Understanding Our Self-Protection Reactions

This blind faith grows because of the physiology of the brain. Our reptilian brain is that part of it that responds to threats and danger. It will take control when it perceives an attack, whether real or imagined. When this part of the brain experiences a threat, immediate effects occur in the body. Our blood chemistry changes, adrenaline is secreted, and the heart rate increases, to name just a few.

We are experiencing what is called the fight-or-flight mechanism, which has benefited us humans since the dawn of time. Either we start running as fast as we can away from danger (say, a huge raptor, or a modern dis-ease), or we use whatever weapon we have at hand (a spear, or a drug vial) to fend off an attack. But in fact there is nowhere safe for us to run, and no creature that we can actually fight. While all this is happening, our reptilian mind has taken control, and therefore our reasoning mind is no longer in the driver's seat. Who *is* in control?

Say that your doctor has just diagnosed you with some life-threatening illness, and suddenly you feel all in a panic. Some psychotherapists[3] have suggested that, when we face a significant and unresolved threat such as cancer, we unconsciously lock onto a deep memory we stored when a young child of the first time we faced a threat without having a parent to help us. We feel unsure of what to do; we are childlike in our responses.

We sometimes are putty in our medical doctor's hands. Under these circumstances, it makes sense that very ill people can easily give up their power and let someone else make all the decisions for them, without ever considering getting a second opinion or seeking out more information to guide them on this tenuous path.

Reaching Out Widely for Help

As we work with our health care practitioners, often putting our bodies and even our very *lives* in their hands, we sometimes have

Consider the Alternatives

In the early 1990s, I visited my parents during my vacation. The night before leaving to go to my own home, I was talking with my mother and father, but I didn't really know what they were trying to tell me. I grew more and more befuddled by the conversation we were having. I could not understand, for the life of me, what they were trying to communicate. Finally I just blurted out, "What's wrong?"

My mother said, "They want to cut your father's legs off."

I started to laugh and, without thinking, shot back, "It's a good thing it's not his head!"

I know this sounds callous and insensitive, but to me this was a preposterous, even outrageous solution to correcting his condition. True, I knew that my father was diabetic and had developed circulation problems. As you might guess, my father, at that time, had little understanding of or faith in the work I had been doing for over 10 years. I didn't always tell him much about it.

I thought for a moment and said, "There are a dozen different options—no, a *thousand* different options—to try before you could even consider any such nonsense." I then went on to name several alternatives (none of my therapies, of course). In the end, my father decided to try intravenous chelation. Since this alternative therapy was not available where they lived in Canada at the time, he went to the United States and did a series of treatments with a medical doctor. Shortly after finishing it he became ill. He was hospitalized and to be willing to draw outside the box, to go beyond the realms of our daily experience, and seek out information from other sources. Doing so is a good deal easier these days, because of the Internet's vast worldwide resources (with health research and study results of all types available online), the help available from a good reference librarian at a public library or community health center, and the vast number of books available that deal with alternative health care.

You have to be discriminating, of course, because not all alternatives are equally effective; some can even be harmful. Seeker, beware! But the information you *do* find can change your life dramatically, without your having to face serious or even invasive medical interventions.

I know that many people will protest; some might say things like, "If it weren't for the medical establishment, I simply wouldn't

---

stayed about a week, with no improvement. One day, my sister, Theresa, asked the staff, "Have you checked his blood sugar levels? He is diabetic." That was the problem: When my father started the IV chelation therapy, he was using about 65 units of insulin a day, but neither he nor any of the medical staff had ever bothered to monitor his blood sugar to see whether there was any change while he was doing the IV chelation process. He was sick because he now only needed about one-third the insulin he had been taking. As a result of improper medical care and self-care, he had been overmedicating himself in the hospital! (Please remember this important point.) When he reduced his insulin to the proper dosage, he began to feel completely normal.

He had also developed ulcers on his feet that pained him terribly. I recommended that he apply melaleuca essential oil, neat, on the sores, and also that he use Stanley Burroughs's Color Therapy (see Chapter 8). My parents soon went to Arizona for the winter, and my father began to take daily walks, and to enjoy them again. He never did have the surgery, nor did he experience any serious problems with his legs ever again. He did have one small toe removed several years later.

Think of the momentous consequences, not only to my father but to the rest of my family, if he had had both legs amputated, which the doctors had recommended as the only course of action. This was avoided completely by just asking for some help from someone with another good idea: me, his son and holistic practitioner.

be alive today." Well, I would challenge that belief in almost every situation when you are dealing with dis-eases. True, if I got into a serious accident in which my bones were broken and I were suffering from internal bleeding or other life-threatening conditions, I would certainly seek emergency medical care. This is where medicine has made tremendous advances. During my recovery at home, I would also want to use all the holistic and alternative tools that I now have at hand, to greatly enhance the effect of any treatment or therapies I received in a hospital or clinic.

Treating Myself

You may have been surprised to read my earlier statement that I have not used a doctor for any medical care since 1980. I have looked after my own body and health, and have used only alternative therapies to treat myself—or, more accurately, to keep myself healthy and avoid the need to consult a physician. You probably know the old adage that says, "A pound of cure is worth an ounce of prevention." Good dis-ease prevention is, in truth, a way toward getting better health for yourself and living a happier, more fulfilling life.

This belief is now getting some serious attention in the business world. IBM is only one of many companies that have begun paying their employees to stay well, rather than waiting to pay for their care when they fall sick or become hospitalized or go out on disability. Several insurance plans are doing something similar. For every dollar the company or plan spends on preventive health programs, they save about three dollars against the need for future care when employees or members fall ill.

I cannot count the times that acquaintances have said to me, with kind of a sneer, "You're doing the Master Cleanse *again*? How often do you do it?" After their next breath, some of them go on to say, almost in spite of themselves, "You always have so much energy and look so healthy all the time!" The surprising thing? That they don't connect the dots.

You might be shocked to read that I generally cleanse for a total of 40, or sometimes even 50, days a year now, and I rarely appear to be or feel unwell. Each cleanse is productive for me and for my unique body system; that many cleanses may not be needed by someone else, with different diet and body chemistry. It should be blatantly obvious to you by now that I do the Master Cleanse regularly, and as a result I am now healthy consistently throughout my life. I also should mention that I do keep an active lifestyle, as well—including exercise, consuming a good diet in moderation, doing work I find fulfilling, and maintaining a positive attitude about life.

Is Conventional Medicine a Slow Learner?

It also appears that conventional medicine, despite its long history of accomplishments, does not learn well from its mistakes. Take the overuse of antibiotics. For many years, antibiotics were prescribed liberally to the general population (as well as to animals and animal products grown for our consumption), and many of them were wonderfully effective. Yet now we have "super bugs" that have become resistant to virtually all drugs designed to eliminate them. Hospital directors around the world are worried to death when they encounter untreatable dis-eases that are impervious to all classes of antibiotics. And now the drug companies are trying to sell you "antiviral" medications. What will they come up with next?

This, to me, is the most telling aspect about how the medical-industrial complex thinks. I see study after study, almost every week, that show a connection between diet and either cancer or a number of other dis-eases.[4] You may recall the Canadian study mentioned in Chapter 1, on the connection between childhood cancer and whether mothers took a prenatal supplement. Anyone with access to a computer can find tens of thousands of articles or extracts on the topic by using a search engine to find specific key words. We know that there is a direct correlation between diet and cancer, but how does medical-industrial complex deal with cancer? Cut, burn, and poison: These are its main tools of intervention. We might profit from taking to heart Albert Einstein's wise remark: "We can't solve problems by using the same kind of thinking we used when we created them."

Did anyone ever get the bright idea that maybe, just maybe, a nutritional therapy might work as well, or even better? It would be heresy if the establishment even tried it.

As only one example of connecting the dots between dis-ease and diet-and-lifestyle, consider the current figures on autism. A staggering 1 in 150 children born in the United States these days is soon afflicted by some form of autism. Thirty years or so ago we didn't even *hear* about such a syndrome. Add one more example: Alzheimer's disease, and how it threatens millions (and perhaps even our financial solvency as a nation). If this is not a case of the canary dying in the coal mine, would somebody please tell me what it is?

The canary is dead, so get the hell out of the mine! *Then find out what's wrong with the air in the mine.*

Whom Can YOU Turn to for Help?

Around the world, people in both developed and underdeveloped countries are facing a range of health problems. To name only a few: bird flu, the threat of a worldwide influenza pandemic, obesity, dis-eases like drug-resistant tuberculosis that are flown across national borders in just hours into a susceptible populace, mad cow disease, e-coli infections of green-leaf crops, serious dis-eases carried in processed meat (causing major recalls), carcasses of pets (euthanized because of dis-ease) recycled into pet food, uncertainties about irradiated food, cloned (bioengineered) plants and animals, gene mixing from one species to another, and on and on. These threats should concern all of us, as consumers and as citizens, not merely as patients and physicians.

But what governmental agency will competently manage such developments and challenges, *and* work to protect us from danger? Can you really trust the Food and Drug Administration, the U.S. Department of Agriculture, and the Department of Health and Human Services to watch out for your interest, down at the personal, human level of you, the consumer? Will you blindly accept their judgments, which are usually influenced by the very corporations and industries they regulate? Do you think they are doing a good enough job for you (remember, they work for you)?

If you do an Internet search of medical journals, you will quickly see that from at least the mid-1970s onward clear evidence has been found of the links between certain foods or nutrients and either the inhibition or promotion of certain dis-eases or illnesses.[5] Although this information has been known to professionals for many years, it has taken decades to come out in the popular media so that we as consumers are able to make informed choices.

How much information about the quality of our foods has been hidden from us as well? I would like to pause here to address the current situation in the food industry. That would take several books, so I will only mention a few of the more impending problems. For starters, consider mad cow disease and how it came about.

Today, the processing of millions of cows for meat and various byproducts creates an enormous volume of unusable carcass parts in America, year after year. Someone in the meat-packing industry must have been watching the 1973 sci-fi movie *Soylent Green,* a movie set in the future. In that future the government dispenses food rations from the Soylent Corp., which produces them in a different color each day—Soylent Red one day, Soylent Yellow the next, and so on. Soylent Green is the newest color to be added to the process. At the end of the movie we find out that Soylent Green is actually made from—wait for it!—human cadavers. The abundance of dead people can now be harvested as a new, plentiful resource to feed those living.

While watching this movie, you have to wonder whether the government bureaucrats and the Soylent Green officials, or today's meat processors, were high or stoned when they got the same bright idea. They just had to process this mass of unusable flesh into palatable pellets, and now they could feed it to the cows. They have taken a vegetarian animal and not only fed it flesh, but also turned it into a cannibal. Is this brilliant, or what? Garbage in, garbage out.

What will they think of next? Let's irradiate food—yeah, that's a good idea. How 'bout we genetically mix the genes from one species into another and make some really cool stuff?

What is happening to our society and our way of life? Who are these people, and why we do we so blindly accept their recommendations? Is nobody out there to oversee and protect us from such insanity?

I urge you to think about the health choices, and food choices, you make today—because tomorrow you may have to pay a price for your poor choices.

I hope that you have become convinced of the need to take charge of your own health, and that of your family. I hope you will vow to cleanse your body regularly, for a variety of persuasive reasons:

Your health plan or HMO is likely not interested in doing it for you, although some are slowly becoming receptive to using preventative medicine.

Your medical doctor has not learned how to do it, and might scoff at it.

You are the person most interested in achieving optimal health for yourself.

Your cleansing might reduce or eliminate a variety of health issues that have been bothering you.

You can reduce your medical costs by avoiding certain illnesses.

You can change the way you eat in the future, but cleansing is one of the few ways that you can address your poor food choices from the past.

You might even save or prolong your life by cleansing regularly.

In the next chapter, you learn how the Master Cleanse works.

CHAPTER 5

What Is the Master Cleanse,

and How Does It Work?

As you now know, the Master Cleanse is one of the most simple, effective, and inexpensive cleansing and healing programs available. The Master Cleanse is a liquid monodiet designed to work with and complement your body's own cleansing and detoxifying processes, and at the same time to effectively nourish your body. It is *not* a fast or a means to starve the body. It is often referred to as a fast, but the true definition of fasting is to drink only water and to starve the body for a given period.

It is true that no solid foods are consumed on the Master Cleanse. This is an absolutely crucial aspect of this diet, for only when we stop the digestive workings of our body can it shift gears to do the now-important task of ridding itself of unnecessary wastes, toxins, or poisons that are creating *dis-ease*. To properly understand how and why the Master Cleanse works, you first must understand how dis-ease manifests in the body. I am using the word dis-ease to describe all conditions or illnesses that can affect the human body.

This chapter will explore both the physical and the emotional dimensions of dis-ease, as prelude to understanding how the Master Cleanse works to detoxify the body and enhance health.

Understanding Dis-ease: A Physical Perspective

Stanley Burroughs, a holistic health practitioner who developed the Master Cleanser and other programs and therapies, believed that all dis-ease conditions that affect the body are caused by *toxemia,* the accumulation of wastes, toxins, or poisons. This buildup is caused by two different mechanisms in our dietary choices:

- Eating devitalized foods
- Consuming foods that have a negative impact on our body

Devitalized foods are those that have been processed to remove or extract their vital ingredients, such as minerals, vitamins, and fiber. Examples are white sugar, white flour, and white rice, to name just a few.

Foods that affect our body negatively include meat and dairy products, artificial foods, preservatives, fried foods, anything containing trans fats, and so on.

Dr. Bernard Jensen, another well-known advocate of cleansing, called the dis-ease mechanism "autointoxification"—or, more to the point, the self-poisoning of the body.[6]

We as a species have evolved, over thousands of years, while eating foods essentially in their whole and natural state. What our distant ancestors ate provided them with the minerals, vitamins, enzymes, fibers, and a host of other essential nutrients to sustain life. But in the last 100 years or so much of our food supply has been processed to remove minerals, vitamins, and fiber to make them look "white" (hence desirable) and to give them a shelf life of years rather than days or weeks. When giant food processing companies wanted more eye appeal and longer shelf life for their products, they started mixing in chemical preservatives, food additives, colorants, artificial flavorings, and a host of other compounds. We have let a group of corporate executives and food scientists (and remember they are just people, not disembodied corporations) increase their profit margins at the expense of our health. Their goal is not our increased health but a rise in their stock price and corporate assets. Their lack of understanding and knowledge of our bodies and its nutritional needs has led them to make many unwise decisions that affect the health of our bodies.

How Our Body Works

Our body is composed of trillions of cells. There are many thousands of specialized types of cells throughout the body, such as bone cells, skin cells, blood cells, nerve cells, brain cells, and so forth. Each of these cell types possesses a very specific structure, shape, function, and chemical makeup. It is this unique chemical makeup that gives each cell all its properties. For all cells to remain healthy, to function perfectly as intended, and to reproduce accurately, they need to be nourished well by our blood, whose task is to carry the necessary building blocks out to the cells.

When your diet is missing certain nutrients, you are actually denying certain types of cells the nutrients they need to function or live. If your cells lack nutrients for a period of time, they will become weak and die (rather than reproduce as new cells). This causes a toxic buildup. It is literally true that *your body is breaking down from the inside out,* some bodies more than others. Of course, we know that a lack of vitamin C causes scurvy, and the lack of certain B vitamins causes beriberi. More recently we have learned that a lack of folic acid can cause birth defects in a newborn child and cervical cancer in a woman. The lack of sufficient calcium in a person's diet has been shown to cause a diminishment of bone strength, which can lead to osteoporosis and resorting to traumatic and expensive repairs such as hip and joint replacement.

We add to this problem by consuming foods that, by their nature, are difficult for us to digest. The leading examples are meat and dairy products. Picture a big hamburger topped with bacon and cheese and egg-based sauces, plus a large milkshake. These two high-protein foods contain no fiber at all, and they also produce unhealthy mucus throughout the digestive system. The lack of fiber and the excess mucus production results in meat and dairy foods moving through our digestive tract at about *one-quarter* the pace of fruit and vegetables. This slow pace ensures that the foods putrefy inside, long before we can eliminate their waste products.

This unfair demand that meat and dairy products place on our body overtaxes our digestive system, making digestion and elimination a burden to the body. No wonder people get tired out, and have to drag themselves through the day until they fall into bed at night! This leads to the eating of white sugar and other processed foods for quick energy, and to consuming stimulants like coffee, tea, carbonated drinks that have no nutritional value whatsoever, and "energy" bars and drinks to get a quick lift or boost of energy.

The Trouble with Processed Foods

Consuming processed foods over a period of time causes a number of problems. To give only a few examples:

- Weakened pancreas (hypoglycemia)
- Destroyed enzymes (which are required for digestion and other functions)
- Reduced fiber (fiber is needed for elimination)
- Accumulation of wastes in the body (toxic buildup)
- Acid formation (leaches out certain essential minerals)

Processed foods weaken the pancreas, causing hypoglycemia. This occurs when the pancreas cannot maintain proper blood sugar levels, which occurs when highly processed foods release sugar into the bloodstream much faster that the body can cope with it. The soaring blood sugar levels stimulate the pancreas into over-production of insulin, which causes the blood sugar levels to plunge. This low energy will motivate the eating of yet *more* sugar to raise blood sugar levels again, and the vicious cycle repeats itself. This is the classic roller-coaster effect caused by processed foods: You eat something for quick energy, your energy spikes up one minute and drops down the next. This stress on the pancreas is compounded by these same white and bleached foods. The minerals and vitamins that have been removed in processing are critically needed for building and maintaining the pancreas. Many metabolic processes that also require these nutrients don't get them in processed food, so are forced to steal them from somewhere else in the body—in essence, robbing from Peter to pay Paul.

The processing and cooking of food also destroys enzymes, compounds that are vital in proper digestion of food and almost every other function in your body. A diet that is low in enzymes or that lacks them completely will push an already stressed pancreas to create digestive enzymes to replace what's missing. It is becoming apparent that the pancreas bears the brunt of attack from a number of poor dietary choices. It is no wonder that some 20 million Americans, many of them children, have diabetes (often linked with obesity, which has its own set of health problems), and the number is growing at a frightening rate.

Fiber is another nutrient that has been removed from many foods. Only recently has fiber been recognized as a critical nutrient, and it is now being added to many products to compensate for the years of its having been removed (go figure!). Think of white bread, white flour, and the like. Fiber has been found to reduce the incidences of certain cancers. It also absorbs acidity as it swells up in the digestive system. Fiber is an indigestible carbohydrate and acts as a bulking agent to enable proper peristalsis to occur. Peristalsis is the wavelike contractions of the muscles throughout the alimentary canal that moves the digesting food, or *chyme,* through the digestive tract. Peristalsis must occur if one is to have regular eliminations of waste from the colon. Fiber deficiency leads to constipation, which in turn starts a host of other problems, and often the consuming of drugs or other products for relief. Diverticulitis is one such problem. A lack of fiber causes people to strain while eliminating. The straining causes pressure on the colon wall, so that pouches or pockets bulge out where there are weaknesses in the wall. These pockets can trap wastes, which further irritate the wall, creating yet more complications.

GOOD TO KNOW

Chyme (pronounced *Kīm*) is the semifluid, homogeneous, creamy or gruel-like material produced as food, water, acids, and digestive enzymes are broken down in the gastric system.

The consumption of foods that leave various accumulations of dis-ease–causing wastes throughout the body is another way in which we make ourselves sick. Meat and dairy products, foods with additives, foods lacking sufficient (or any) fiber, and hydrogenated fats (including trans fats) are the main culprits in this grouping.

Acid Formation

A common link exists among most, perhaps all, foods that are toxic to the body—they are acid forming. Most of the foods that people eat in the Western world are acid forming, which means that when the digestion process is complete the waste products left over are acidic. One way in which our body compensates for this high acidity is to leach specific neutralizing minerals (such as calcium, magnesium, and potassium) out of the tissues. This process, if allowed to happen unchecked, will lead to other deficiencies and problems that soon have to be dealt with.

When we are in a healthy state our blood acidity reads about 7.3 to 7.4 on the pH scale; 7.0 is neutral on the scale. As the number increases, you become more alkaline; as the number decreases, you become more acid.

If you eat a diet high in acid-forming foods, such as meat, dairy, processed foods, and dried beans and grains, your body starts to become overacid. This creates an entirely different and undesirable chemistry in the body. (Try getting the chemistry wrong when baking a cake, or developing film in a tray of chemicals in a photo lab. You'll get and ingestion, or crummy photos.)

Candida

As an example, *Candida albicans* is a yeast, or fungus, that lives in the colon with hundreds of other organisms that help to break down and prepare waste products to be eliminated. This intestinal organism lives in a delicate balance with these many other intestinal flora. If the colon becomes overly acidic, *Candida* can grow into an overabundance, just like too much ivy growing up a brick wall, and thus become a menace to your health.

One of *Candida*'s jobs is to make your waste biodegradable. When someone dies, as the body decays from a lack of oxygen it quickly becomes acidic and so the *Candida* grows rapidly, helping to make the body biodegradable—that is, ready to return its components to the earth (barring the use of embalming fluids).

But in the living body, problems arise as your body becomes increasingly acid from your diet. The *Candida* and other organisms will start to grow in this newfound environment. Thrush (candidiasis), yeast infections, dandruff, nail infections, and dozens of other symptoms are direct outgrowths of overacidity. Not only are these many different microorganisms literally living off your body—in other words, *eating you alive*—but also they are consuming your body's supply of glucose, fats, and proteins. Added to this, they secrete into the body their waste byproducts, called mycotoxins and exotoxins, which are another form of acid waste (or let's call it "toxic waste").

When you open the door to such microorganisms, it is as if you welcome someone into your home who eats up your food and defecates everywhere and dirties everything in sight, with no consideration for you at all.

If you follow the traditional allopathic medical practice, you would use a prescription drug (in the form of a manufactured pill or liquid) to attack and kill the offending organisms. At first this makes sense. But later on you learn that these drugs often kill many of the positive intestinal organisms ("good bacteria") that aid in digestion, causing various side effects. Using logic, when the environment of our body gets out of balance by becoming overly acid, then we simply need to alkalize our body.

From this we can make the obvious conclusion that we need to eat a mostly alkaline diet. Many nutritionists and health scientists suggest that, for an optimal diet, 80 percent of our food intake would be alkaline and 20 percent would be acidic.

Now, to better understand how toxemia creates the many illnesses that the medical field treats (whether for ill or good), you need to learn a few things about your colon, and how dis-ease generally starts there.

Organs of Elimination

You probably know that your colon is an organ of elimination. It is about 5 feet long, and 2½ to 3 inches in diameter. It ascends the right side of the abdomen and stops underneath the liver. It then transverses from the right to left to just under the spleen. It then descends along the left side of the body to the sigmoid colon and then to the rectum and out to the anus. The colon is essentially a long membrane that allows excess moisture and a small amount of minerals and vitamins to be extracted from the chyme and thence to be absorbed into the bloodstream. What it leaves is eliminated as a bowel movement from the body.

In addition to the colon, there are four other organs of elimination:

- Skin
- Lungs
- Kidneys
- Sinuses

The largest organ of elimination is the lungs. Many people may be surprised by this statement, insisting that the skin is the largest such organ. But each lung, with its minute sacs, or alveoli, contains from 250 to 375 square feet of surface area, while the skin has only some 20 square feet of surface area. True, the skin is the largest in terms of mass or weight, yet the lungs expel more waste byproducts than the skin does. By this measure, the lungs rank first, the skin second, the colon third, and (depending on the individual) the kidneys and sinuses are a tie, being either fourth or fifth. As you read further, you will learn that many problems in these other organs of elimination arise from a colon's being unable to manage its own waste disposal adequately.

Foods' Impact on the Colon

Directly or indirectly, many foods have a tremendous impact on the colon's health, some for good, some for ill. The main culprits are foods low in fiber (or completely lacking in it), foods high in fat and low in nutrient content (that is, most processed foods), and foods that are acid forming. Such foods act as an irritant that causes the body to respond by producing mucus, which acts as a buffer to lessen their negative impact on the body. This excess mucus impedes an already slow transit time through the digestive tract caused by poor or no fiber in these foods. This problem is further compounded by certain foods' acidic nature. This overly acid environment now becomes a breeding ground for yeast, molds, fungi, bacteria, and parasites.

Now we have this overacid, slow-moving slurry passing through the colon like a slow train on a side track. As it slowly progresses it putrefies, thereby playing host to a number of organisms multiplying within it. To these problems you now add the excess mucus that the body creates, as well as the related problems of poorly digested food, impaired peristalsis, the emotional stress that can result, and dehydration. Constipation is an obvious outcome of these many problems. It should come as no surprise that the laxative industry sells billions of dollars worth of products to an ill-informed and naive public, who are treating the *symptoms* rather than addressing the problem.

When the body contains an excess weight of waste products in the colon, another problem results and has a dramatic negative effect on the body. The colon starts to droop or sag as gravity pulls down on this excess waste and becomes *prolapsed*, or out of its usual position. This further impedes proper flow through the colon, causing even more constipation.

Have you ever wondered what might be in someone's bloated or inflated belly? I have seen many X-rays that are almost unbe-

> ### Cancer and Pregnancy
>
> My former wife had cervical cancer. We were told that she had to undergo a hysterectomy in the next few days. We chose instead to use the Master Cleanse, Color Therapy, and Vita-Flex therapies, and to try Louise L. Hay's teachings to deal with specific emotional issues, as our therapies of choice. My wife then had our first child nine months later, with her cancer gone and no medical intervention or procedures used. Less than a year later, our second child was born. We were in the hospital for only 1 hour and 20 minutes before our child was delivered (weighing almost 11½ pounds). My wife checked herself out in less than 1 hour and 30 minutes after delivering our son.

lievable, showing colons in extremely distorted and twisted positions, with strictures and ballooning throughout their length. It is as if someone came into your house when you were away and bent all your drainpipes. In women, a prolapsed colon becomes a specific problem to the reproductive system, as the colon, now overburdened, slips down a bit and starts to poison the surrounding organs and tissues.

A drooping colon that lies on a woman's ovaries, uterus, and bladder can provoke many undesirable conditions of the reproductive system, including endometriosis, PMS, yeast infections, incontinence, and even infertility. (See illustrations on page 120.) I have seen about a 50 percent success rate with formerly infertile women being able to become pregnant after completing several Master Cleanses and receiving a series of colon lifts.

It makes sense that this slow-moving sticky, acidic, dehydrated, and putrefied material trying to make its way through the length of the colon is host to many organisms, including parasites. Because the chyme is extremely sticky, it starts to adhere to the colon wall. We know this happens, because if it didn't then people wouldn't need to use toilet paper after evacuation.

This continual accumulation of sticky waste over many years, even a lifetime, can lead to several pounds of old fecal material residing in the colon alone. You might well be wondering why, if this is so prevalent, don't more people know about this condition? And why doesn't medicine address this problem as well?

Many holistic health practitioners believe that well over 90 percent of all conditions start in the colon and spread throughout the rest of the body. I often explain to clients that the colon becomes somewhat akin to a toxic waste site—even worse, your own colon is a waste dump that you take with you wherever you go and however fancily you're dressed.

My own experience with the Master Cleanse was quite enlightening, because I lost nine pounds the first time I did it. At least half of this weight loss—or, as I now like to say, "waste loss"—was old debris that had been impacted in my colon, along with a lot of mucus. You might take a moment right now to look down at your waist line and wonder how much waste is stored in your colon. The bigger your waist size, usually the bigger the waste mound inside.

I hope that it is becoming evident to you that eating the wrong things can lead to serious conditions within your colon. Let's now look at how this creates dis-ease throughout the rest of the body.

The continual irritation of the colon's lining by an acidic layer causes inflammation and loss of tissue integrity. Such irritation can go on to cause what is known as "leaky gut syndrome," also called "leaky bowel syndrome." This occurs when some of the contents of the colon leak into the abdominal cavity. The extra acidity affects the porous-like nature of the colon wall, which allows moisture and mineral content to pass through it and into the bloodstream. That membrane will become so porous as to allow yeasts, molds, fungi, bacteria, parasites, and waste to get into the bloodstream. The bloodstream, laden with toxicity, transports these toxins throughout the entire body, just like a river carrying silt after a thunder shower. Just as the river will deposit the silt wherever the river bends or slows, so the bloodstream will slow down where stress is being experienced in the body.

My own analogy for this description of dis-ease, and how modern medicine treats dis-ease, goes like this: Let's say you walk into your bathroom to find your bathtub overflowing. Instead of turning off the faucet and removing the stopper, you grab a mop and start mopping up the water, wringing it out in the toilet. After several hours of this, since the water continues to flow, you decide to call for help and hire someone to do this job for you. Finally, after a week or two, and from your rented hotel room (clinic or hospital room), you find a plumber (doctor) so that he might install a drain (intervene medically) on the bathroom floor (your poor body). Clearly there is a much simpler way to correct this problem. Step #1 is to shut off the tap; in other words, *stop feeding your illness.* Step #2 is to pull the plug, or *start eliminating* through the process of cleansing and detoxification.

Now I will throw one more wrench into the metaphor. Many years ago I read about a study done by a physician on the long-term effects of appendectomies that were routinely done on patients, whether they needed them or not. The study found that patients whose appendix had been removed experienced a 50 percent higher risk of developing colon cancer. It was Stanley Burroughs's opinion that the appendix had a function—to secrete

Colon Lift to Reach a Healthy Condition

One of my friends referred his father to me for treatment. I monitored him while he did a Master Cleanse for 10 days. On Day 3 or so, I suggested that he come in for a prolapsed colon lift. This is a treatment that lifts or moves the colon back up into its natural position. I believe that well over 95 percent of the population above the age of 20 are prolapsed. The excess weight in the colon and the lack of muscle tone in the abdominal area are the main causes of this condition.

My friend's father, who I will call "Bill," expressed some hesitation and skepticism about my simple technique. I further explained the necessity for this procedure and the positive results he could expect, including maximizing the benefits of the Master Cleanse. Bill said that he was still unsure that he needed the process and asked how he would positively know that he would be benefited. I suggested that he go to his doctor and get an X-ray after receiving a barium enema into his colon; this would show the colon's condition position. As it happened, Bill never returned and I never followed up with him. As life would have it, about two years later my friend got engaged and I ran into Bill during the wedding. I had not seen him for two years or so. With-a thin lubricant where the small intestine met with the colon (at the ileocecal valve) to allow the chyme to transit the colon more quickly. How many people do *you* know whose appendix has been taken out?

Up to this point, I have only been talking about the physical aspects that affect your health. But now let's consider the mental/emotional realm, which is also part of our body system. We must go there because some of you might be saying such things as: "I eat well." Or "I am a vegetarian and don't eat any processed food." Or maybe "I am completely a raw foodist." But even these practices may not be enough.

Haven't we all heard about folks who ate poorly, drank often, maybe even smoked up a storm, were widowed young, and proceeded to live to 100—longer than many other people who lived an outwardly healthier lifestyle? What you may not recognize or notice is that stress may be the dominant factor or influence on the state of your health.

out hesitation or a hello Bill said to me, "I got that X-ray you suggested." It took me a second or so, then I asked, "What did the doctor say?" Bill responded, "He said it was normal." I said, "Did you view the X-ray yourself?" Bill replied, "Yes." I asked, "Did you see a big U-shape in the middle?" Again Bill replied, "Yes." I said, "Bill, that is a prolapsed colon. It should not look like a big U at all. It should look like the diagram I showed you." Bill said, "The doctor told me that I was normal and that what you said was a lot of hot air."

Now, I agree with some of what that doctor told Bill. Yes, a colon such as his *may be* considered a normal colon today, if by "normal" you mean average or usual. But is it natural? And does this normal condition create a state of optimal health, or of failing health?

When I started my alternative practice, little was known about colon health and the effect of diet on the incidence of cancer. In 1980, as I was intensifying my health and body studies, the statistics stated that about one person in four got cancer, a rate that was considered the norm. Today, however, the norm is an alarming *one person in three*. "Normal" or "usual" is not what I am looking for. Instead, my goal is to help create what is "natural" or healthy both to our mind and to our body.

Letting It Go

At one time my sister worked in a senior citizens center, taking care of the residents. She preferred to work the midnight shift so that she could care for her two children during the day. It happened that more people died at night, and she was required to clean the body before it was transported to the funeral home. One day she asked me about the black, tarry substance with a horrific odor that passed from the bodies after death. It should be clear to you what it is at this point in the book. It seems that we humans will not let go of all our waste until after we die. Why? Maybe because we are so unwilling to let go of our own shit!

The Effects of Stress

When you are experiencing a long-term indefinable stress, your body begins many different chemical, hormonal, and metabolic processes, all without your permission. You may be experiencing the fight-or-flight response, discussed in Chapter 4. Actually, rarely is the stress you are experiencing all that threatening. Your stress may be coming from your worry about making the rent this month, global warming over the next few decades, or keeping your job at least until your children are grown.

While there may be no life-threatening adversary staring you in the face, no real attack that you need to flee from, if this stress remains unresolved for a long time the effects on your body can be dramatic. For example, after about two minutes of stress the digestive system slows and may even stop until the situation is resolved. (Think about misplaced road rage, which now and then results in a drive-by shooting and a fatality.) Even with the best diet, any stress at all will have some impact on the health of your body.

Stress is a condition that starts in the conscious mind and almost always manifests as a feeling in the body. When left unchecked or resolved, it becomes an unconscious state in the mind, which then settles into the body's tissues and cells. It's similar to working on your computer with 10 websites open, downloads happening, backups and virus checks going on in the background, and your computer has slowed down to a crawl. In the physical body, this unconscious state, if left unchecked for too long, will create the experience of a dis-ease or discomfort, functioning much like an alarm to alert the mind and wake it up to take corrective action.

In my own experience, whenever I failed to express myself comfortably within one of my relationships, guess what? I would have a sore throat every month. With stress some people have a herpes outbreak, or shingles, and on and on. Even if you eat well, your body is affected by your thoughts. No one is immune to the effects of stress or worry.

Understanding Dis-ease: An Emotional Perspective

Until this point I have addressed dis-ease mostly from a physical level—at the level of the body. Most people first identify illness by the physical symptoms that cause them discomfort or pain. I believe that all illness starts in the mind first and then manifests physically as a symptom or series of symptoms. These symptoms—which can be pain or discomfort of any sort—are simply the warning bells and lights, just like on the dashboard of your car. When my car's engine overheats, a light flashes and an alarm sounds. This means that I should slow down, then stop, and address what is wrong.

With our physical bodies a problem occurs when we do not understand our warning signals and continue to live our life the same way, without taking corrective action. It is obvious that when you continue to ignore the warnings and drive your car this way, it will overheat and eventually destroy the engine. Remember the adage: If you always do what you have always done, you will always get what you have always gotten.

How Our Mind Works

To more fully understand the connection between your mind and body, you have to understand how the mind works within the body.

Researchers have found that with each emotion or feeling we experience, we produce compounds or molecules in the brain that are released into the bloodstream. These molecules, called neuropeptides, are composed of two or more amino acids and are produced by neurons. They are the intercellular messengers to the body. They deliver chemical messages that tell the body, in effect, what the mind is feeling, whether it's a happy memory of a loved one, or the yummy smell of a favorite dinner, or the joy elicited by hearing a piece of music. The function of these neuropeptides is to slide into receptor sites on the walls or membrane of the cells throughout our entire body.

The very shape and function of these molecules are akin to how a key slides effortlessly into a lock, but only one specific lock. This lock, or the receptor site of the cell, is far more sophisticated than a metal lock, because it can read the shape of a molecule and from this derive information to make the cell function in highly specific ways. It is as if your consciousness is being chemically spread throughout your body to every cell, by means of these neuropeptides. **Mind over Body.** These neuropeptides control mood, regulate energy levels, suppress or cause inflammation, and govern body weight. They even regulate the immune system, and do much, much more.

You can appreciate this process by remembering how you felt when you were deeply in love. Your body felt lighter as if you were floating on air, you had more energy, you seemed to need less sleep, maybe you even ate less, you had less pain in your body or even no pain at all. Now compare that to how your body feels today when you get depressed or angry. You may feel heavy, grumpy, sleepy, and sad—or full of fire, full of rage and vindictiveness. You have a completely different experience in your body than the feeling you had of being in love. This difference in your feelings between winning and losing at poker, or in a pick-up basketball game, is another apt comparison.

Close your eyes and imagine biting into a lemon. Did your mouth salivate in anticipation? The point is that what you think doesn't have to be real to have an effect on your entire being. Your unconscious mind cannot distinguish between your present experience and your imagination—nor, for that manner, can it tell the difference between the past, present, and future. The unconscious mind takes everything you think, hear, speak, and do, and accepts it without judgment or discernment. Therefore, it is vital that you take care where you put your mind, and what you choose to expose it to.

How Our Receptor Brain Cells Learn and Adapt

In the brain, the receptor sites on the cellular wall are varied, to accept many different types of peptides. When a given cell starts to become inundated with the same neuropeptide, as the cell reproduces itself it will become more and more specialized to receive that molecule or that emotion. This is an important point, as the consequences can be significant.

We can be highly adaptive to our environment, adjusting to its positive or negative influence. Any new constant influence becomes a normalized state for the body in response to an experience. If we choose to feel angry in response to many life experiences, our brain will create many "angry" neuropeptides that run out as chemical messengers to the body's trillions of cells. The cells that are exposed constantly to these "angry" molecules will start to program more and more receptor sites to fit this compound as the cell reproduces itself. Thus, the cells are first programming and then creating a new wave of cells that will be less receptive to the "happy" neuropeptides or any other neuropeptides and the emotional states they carry. This process also creates havoc in your body when it is angry all the time; high blood pressure is just one example of the bad effects.

The chemical industry always keeps an eye on us. While it has greatly improved the quality of life in many areas, it has fallen short in other significant areas. The chemical industry produces tens of thousands of new chemical compounds every year, some of which are toxic to our body. Many personal care products contain numerous synthetic compounds structured to fit into receptor sites on the cells but not to be released (as in "I've fallen and I can't get up").

This is not always a good thing, because then these cells can no longer function properly and become a burden to the rest of the body. It is as if someone went throughout a factory handcuffing the employees to their machines, one by one. I recently heard a medical doctor speaking about blocked receptor sites in cells and an apparent related increase in the incidence of type II diabetes. When receptor sites for insulin are impaired, the cells cannot absorb sufficient glucose.

It is evident that the body is a self-regulating mechanism and will take every step possible to maintain wellness. But its self-regulation for optimal health can easily be overridden by a constant diet of unhealthy food, or even by a daily pattern of negative and unhealthy thoughts.

The average person has some forty to fifty thousand thoughts each and every day. Most occur in our unconscious mind, where they run freely in and out, without affecting our behavior too much. The majority of these thoughts run like an endless-loop cassette tape around and around in our minds. It would be great if we could consciously examine every thought and separate them into two piles. The first pile would be for thoughts that uplift us or advance our lives—thoughts such as "I am wonderful" / "Life is great" / "I really love my job" / "I have awesome friends" / "My partner is truly loving." In the second pile are thoughts or beliefs that weigh us down and prevent our life from being as wonderful and creative as it can be—thoughts like "Life is just a struggle" / "I don't want to be sick" / "Something bad is always going to happen" / "I am stupid." If you could then compare the size and height of both piles, I believe you could clearly tell how you experience life and how healthy you are by which pile was the largest.

A study was done with kittens placed in an environment that had no vertical lines. When the kittens had matured to a certain age, they were placed into another environment. This new environment had vertical lines, such as posts, that the cats could not seem to see, so they would continually bump into them.

Feelings of Self-Worth

One afternoon, I was driving my daughter and one of her friends home from school. As I listened to the girls talk, it became apparent that her friend was feeling very low self-esteem. After dropping her friend off at her home I asked my daughter if her friend spoke about herself by saying things like "I am stupid." My daughter replied, "How did you know?" It was clear to me that someone had been telling this young girl, ever since she was a small child, that she was stupid. So she now acted as if she was indeed stupid. She was becoming what she had been programmed by others to be.

It becomes clear that the thoughts we think affect us and the thoughts we share with others can have a long and lasting impact.

One of my clients, who is a dentist, told me that every day in dentistry school the same person stood up and said, "Life is a bitch and then you die" It might have made people laugh, but such constant negative programming will have a consequence unless you delete it from your mind. This individual was complaining that life was most unjust and that it was unfair that all these bad things happened in their life.

The Body as an Extension of the Mind

The day that the Beatles' John Lennon was shot outside his apartment in Manhattan, I watched a TV program about his life. In one of the clips Lennon was saying that people who believed in pacifism, or the peace movement, or nonviolence were always shot. He mentioned the Kennedys, Martin Luther King, Jr., and Gandhi. (Later, one of my clients told me that he had read about John Lennon and learned that he was somewhat obsessed about guns.)

One Friday night several years later, while watching videos on television, I heard an audio clip of Lennon made just hours before he was shot. In it he was talking about people being shot for their political or religious beliefs and nonviolence. Do you see a connection? I know that this may trigger disbelief for many people at this point, but please bear with me. Many physicists now say that the nature of reality is a result of our beliefs or perceptions. In fact, to overcome biases or personal perceptions, double-blind studies are typically done, so that the awareness of an individual would not affect the outcome of the test.

David Suzuki, a well-known Canadian environmentalist and TV personality, spoke about a study performed to determine whether the mind could affect machines. The test was done on a simple machine that consisted of a plywood sheet lying on an angle with barriers on both sides and also at the bottom of the board. Near the bottom were 10 holes big enough for Ping-Pong balls to fall through. Each hole was numbered 1 through 10, and a collection bag was attached to each hole. The experimenters then rolled a number of balls from the top down toward the holes. When all the balls had fallen through the holes, the bags were collected and the number of balls counted that had gone into each hole. Researchers charted this information onto a graph and found an obvious bell curve showing that the largest number

Laughter Lifts Pain

A friend of mine attended a small presentation on live blood analysis in someone's home. A drop of blood from one of the participants was placed on a glass slide, which was placed under a dark-field microscope to magnify blood cells to the size of saucers when viewed on a TV monitor. The particular sample of blood showed the red blood cells sticking together, as if stacked like pancakes, making long snake-like patterns in the surrounding plasma. This indicated a problem in the contributor's blood, since the cells should be free-floating in the plasma. While watching this on the TV screen someone told a joke that made the blood donor laugh quite hard. Even though the donor and her blood were no longer in contact, the blood shown on the screen changed immediately and the blood cells separated from each other. It seems that our mind really *can* affect our body, even when it is outside our self.

On the same topic, Norman Cousins, long-time editor of *Saturday Review*, made famous his use of laughter to heal himself from a painful and debilitating illness that was thought to be incurable. (In fact, he lived for 26 years after his doctors diagnosed his heart condition.) As he was changing his lifestyle, he decided he would watch funny movies and amusing television programs to make himself laugh. That gave him respite from his pain for many years. I guess he found out that you can't laugh yourself to death.

of balls went into the center holes, while the least number of balls fell into holes near either edge.

Here is where it gets interesting. Next, a glass window was placed between the test device and a participating observer, and as the balls were rolled down he or she was asked to think "right" (direction). The bags were collected and the balls counted and rolled down again. Then the observer was asked to think "left," and the balls were counted. The results were once more charted. After several people did the test, the results were charted. Observers who were asked to think "right" had the bell curve move the same way, while those asked to think "left" had their bell curve move in that direction. This is an amazing but telling experiment that should raise many questions about the power of the mind.

So now the question is, "Why should I do the Master Cleanse if I can think myself well?" Addressing dis-ease at the physical level is much easier than addressing thought patterns. The body is more accessible than the mind. We can more easily control what we put in our mouths than in our minds. By treating our body we can easily and more quickly see or feel the results.

The body is an extension of the mind. The mind is made up of both our conscious awareness and our unconscious awareness, working together. Here's where it gets tricky. We learn more by the age of 2 or 3 than we do the rest of our lives, and most of what we learn comes from our role models—our parents. The rest comes from church or temple, school, the state, the media, the surrounding culture, and whatever other influences we are exposed to. These many influences shape the way we think, feel, and live our lives, and also affect whether our lives are based on truth or lies. For example, when I ask someone their age, where they live, or what their name is, they do not have to think about the answers. This information is now in the unconscious mind for easy access, as is all the rest of the stuff that someone taught or told you. Now, what's inside your head might not always be working in your best interests. Most people don't really know what is going on in there. But there is a way to find out.

What's going on in our body is determined by those pesky neuropeptides, which sometimes cause havoc in your body but which are really a blessing (and, of course, a necessity for living). The neuropeptides make the body respond specifically to each and every thought, belief, and emotion. The body and its symptoms then become a road map to the destination of the mind. You have to know how to read the signs, go around the blind curves, to understand what the unconscious mind is thinking.

We now need a legend for the body. It turns out that it has been available for more than 20 years, in the book *You Can Heal Your Life*, by Louise L. Hay. One chapter in the book lists conditions or problems of the body, next to another list of the most probable thoughts or beliefs that created the conditions or symptoms. It also provides a number of affirmations, or positive thoughts, to help readers reprogram their mind and heal their body.

Here is one of Hay's examples:

Problem: Constipation
Probable Cause: Refusing to release old ideas. Stuck in the past. Sometimes stinginess.
New Thought Pattern: As I release the past, the new and fresh and vital enter. I allow life to flow through me.

I'd like to add one comment to Hay's example. What is so great about this tool is that we can change ourselves at the very core of our being if we choose to, because we have Free Will.

Affirming Life

I was treating a woman in her 70s, who told me that in the past she had had pancreatic cancer. I asked her what she had done by way of treatment. She replied, to my utter astonishment, that she did positive affirmations 12 hours a day for several weeks! She went on to say that her doctor had never known anyone else to recover from her type of pancreatic cancer. While I cannot confirm this story, I believe it to be possible. If true, then at least in her case many hours a day of fixed, positive attention in the appropriate way could very well heal the body. How many people do you know who would even consider such an endeavor? Probably not many.

GOOD TO READ: LET THE SUN SHINE IN

I myself and a number of my clients and colleagues have gotten a great many things of value from the writings of Louise L. Hay. Her inspiring and supportive books continue to be popular. Favorite books cover ways to heal your life, work through patterns of co-dependence, better understand the mental causes of illness, release anger, and love yourself more.

How the Master Cleanse Works

Now that we understand the problem of dis-ease from both the physical and the emotional realms, the solution will be much easier to understand and appreciate. The solution is simple: cleanse. No news-headline here: *The best cleanse I have found in my long practice is the Master Cleanse.* It will detoxify the body's tissues, break down old wastes to be eliminated, and clean the receptor sites of cells. It will do these chores effectively, while still assisting in the regeneration of unhealthy tissues and cells throughout the entire body.

As you drop your old waste into the toilet, in a sense you are also dropping your old thoughts and belief systems down the drain. But you still need to firmly let go of these beliefs. Releasing them is more readily accomplished when you are the proud owner of a body that both looks and feels better. If you were driving in a NASCAR race, would you rather be at the wheel of a car with balding tires, poor suspension, and a motor barely running on five cylinders...or would you prefer a souped-up, shiny, turbo-charged, well-lubricated speedster in the best possible running condition?

Most people have to experience the Master Cleanse first-hand before they will believe that it can produce amazing results. After you do one or more cleanses, depending on your physical condition and other factors, your body will, in all likelihood, change and become healthier. This will give you the opportunity to then start to change your negative thoughts and patterns as well, which in turn will support you in your goal of staying healthier— and so the cycle continues. This cyclical effect may also change for the better some of the ways you think about the world and your community, and may even enhance your spiritual state.

Detoxification

To stay alive, our body has few but highly specific needs—oxygen, water, food, and rest. For the body to remain alive and healthy, the quality of these needs has to be of the highest order. When these needs are not met, a certain amount of stress develops, which then starts a downward negative effect on the body's health. This leads to illness or dis-ease. There is only one way to properly address this problem: to cleanse or detoxify the body, while at the same time feeding it the best possible nutrients so that it can regenerate itself in a healthy manner. Cleansing the body down to the level of the cells requires that the digestive process be almost completely shut down for repairs. In normal living, the digestive process's constant need to be running can consume some 25 percent of the body's energy. In fact, digestion is such a complicated process that when scientists tried to mimic the body's digestive system without using heat and pressure it required several rooms full of equipment.

But now it seems that we have a bit of a contradiction here: How can we feed the body (keep its engines going) and detoxify it (shut off its engines for cleaning) at the same time? We need a program that uses the least amount of digestive energy expenditure, is highly nutritious, and can cleanse the body of any and all wastes with great efficiency.

How Our Food Gets Processed

Everything we eat must be broken down into a liquid-soluble form by a number of chemical and mechanical processes that take place. Our body reduces these solid foods to simple compounds so that they can pass through the small intestinal wall into the bloodstream, to be sent all around the body and absorbed where needed.

The Master Cleanse consists of a liquid monodiet that, in itself, is very simple to digest. It contains an abundance of nutrients in a liquid-soluble form, together with all the enzymes necessary for digestion and other necessary functions. Happily, this low workload for the digestive system also creates another positive outcome: We can now assimilate more of what we are eating—or, when on the Master Cleanse, what we are drinking.

This diminished burden on the digestive system frees up not only energy but also enzymes, which can be utilized to heal the body. This is what puts the body into the overdrive state that you experience while on the Master Cleanse. This is deep cleansing indeed—often an extraordinary experience that a few people find difficult to cope with. Some folks start a cleanse not believing that they truly deserve to feel well, so to shut down that feeling they go off and eat a peanut butter and jelly sandwich. That wonderful experience is then short-lived and they feel like they are dying. How do I know? Because they call me, asking what they can do to stop the pain.

Another byproduct of the cleanse is feeling more relaxed and calm. The body also becomes less rigid. Together, these two effects add up to a net energy gain. I'll tell you a funny/wonderful story: My teacher took the training from Stanley Burroughs to prove he was a fraud. In a 60-day period he did the Master Cleanse for a total of 56 days. He ended up losing 60 pounds, he passed a tumor, his allergies went away, his back problem cleared up, *and* while on the Master Cleanse he was vigorously running 10 miles a day! He considered all these results to be proof that Burroughs' monodiet worked, in significant ways. (See his testimonial and photos in Chapter 13.)

Autolysis and Enzymes

Many people considering doing a cleanse ask how they can possibly survive on such a simple diet. They think it would be like going into the desert to starve. In fact, studies have shown that people can live up to 100 days without eating any food at all. The longest I have known anyone to do the Master Cleanse is 372 consecutive days (far longer than most people will want to stay on it). This simple diet is packed with a number of nutrients that will feed the body and energetically start the body in self-cleansing.

In the next chapter, I will talk more about the ingredients. But for now, it's good to know that our body has an amazing recycling plant always running within it. The recycling of nutrients within the body is called *autolysis*, which literally means "digestion of the self" by self-produced enzymes. As only one example, your body will recycle 80 percent of the protein it takes in.

This process of autolysis is managed by *enzymes* in the body. Enzymes are proteins that act as catalysts to regulate and assist in chemical reactions. Their job is to assemble complex substances from simpler compounds and also to disassemble complex substances into simpler compounds. Enzymes will both create proteins from amino acids and, conversely, make amino acids from protein. They assist in breaking down fats throughout the body. They also break down cells, both the healthy and the unhealthy ones, to suit the body's needs. Enzymes carry out innumerable functions throughout the body; a body that does not have enough enzymes cannot survive.

The enzymes in lemon juice, an ingredient in the Master Cleanse, are extremely sensitive, as are all enzymes found in citrus foods. These enzymes may only be vital for 10 minutes outside the fruit. They can be destroyed by heat, light, and oxygen. So, for the Master Cleanse to work at its best, you should not heat your lemonade above 118°F, nor warm it up in a microwave oven, nor premix a gallon and let it sit for a day or two. You want to drink the *live* enzymes.

SHUN THE MICROWAVE

Microwaving the lemonade, or any food, depletes its life energy. Microwaving makes vitamins and minerals useless or decreases their nutrients, renders protein worthless, causes fruits and vegetables to be harder to digest, and makes food acid-forming.[7]

When you starve a body by fasting, the complete lack of nutrition forces the process of autolysis to become extremely selective. Because all tissues are made up of nutrients from the food we eat, all our tissues, whether healthy or unhealthy ones, become a reserve that is accessed in times of need. The tissues or cells most vulnerable to autolysis are either dead or dying, and will be used first. While the body is being further starved, autolysis will eat up to 97 percent of its fat and then go on to consume other specific organs, then muscle tissue, and so on. In a kind of self-protective mode, the brain, heart, and spinal cord experience the least amount of autolysis, or about 3 percent. Unhealthy tissues such as tumors can sometimes be dissolved by the process of autolysis. It stands to reason that, if your body can create something, why can it not eliminate it, too?

During the Master Cleanse, the process of autolysis becomes extraordinarily streamlined. When the cleanse is done properly—that is, when you consume a sufficient number of glasses a day of the lemonade mixture—the body will be receiving enough calories to maintain a high metabolic rate. The body is, in fact, not being starved but is being assisted to break down that which is no longer useful or functional to it. Lemon juice has an ionic makeup similar to digestive juices, and on the cleanse it can work uncompromised, without having other foods present in the digestive system competing and disrupting the cleansing process.

Our Body's Water

When born, our body may be as much as 90 percent water. As we mature, our water content will lessen to about 70 percent, but in the case of some elderly it can drop even to 60 percent. When we fail to take in enough water every day, many metabolic functions are inhibited and nutrients are absorbed incompletely, both of which significantly slow the removal of wastes from our body. Old waste in the colon putrefies and will also dehydrate. Then we often resort to stool softeners, because our stool has become so dry it will not easily exit the body. Dehydration, in turn, stresses the kidneys, causes headaches, and even affects blood pressure.

The Master Cleanse is very effective in reversing all these symptoms by the simple process of proper hydration of the body through drinking 6 to 12 glasses a day of the lemonade mixture. I recommend that people drink at least 8 glasses of lemonade per day. Many people choose to drink water as well during the cleanse.

Acidity

You may be wondering how to deal with the accumulation of acidity throughout the body's tissues. The lemon and cayenne pepper in the Master Cleanse are extremely alkalizing to the body as it neutralizes acids. After the tissues have been neutralized, the water will flush their acidity out into the various organs of elimination. The decreased acidity will reduce inflammation and swelling. Swelling is caused when the body is pushed past its limits of toxicity and retains excess fluids to dilute the body's acidity.

The Master Cleanse will also help to oxygenate the tissues and blood. Lemon is high in oxygen, and the cayenne pepper both stimulates the heart and thins the blood.

Together, the lemon and cayenne break up and loosen mucus that has been holding irritants and poisons in various areas of the body. I recall treating one client when, halfway through our session, she had to run to the bathroom. When she returned several minutes later her eyes were as big as saucers. I asked her what had happened and she replied, "I have just passed several pounds of mucus!"

As a body becomes more alkaline, its oxygen levels increase and mucus is eliminated. This creates an environment that is hostile to parasites and various microorganisms, which cannot live in such a home. The complete elimination of parasites can be a lengthy process with just the Master Cleanse alone.

The laxative that is taken as a component of the cleanse will cause peristalsis in the colon, where the majority of toxicity resides. This will eliminate what is being freed up within the colon.

In addition, the lemon and cayenne break up and loosen wastes in the body. The water flushes toxins out of the tissues and hydrates and loosens old dehydrated wastes in the colon. The laxative then purges the body of what it no longer needs or finds useful. The other four organs of elimination (skin, lungs, kidneys, and sinuses) also will function at a higher capacity when the colon stops dumping its excesses into the bloodstream that they share with it. At the same time, the diminished burden of wastes and the safe near-shutdown of the digestive system both make it much easier for the body to regenerate and heal itself.

But Aren't We All Different?

Once my clients learn the details of the Master Cleanse and its benefits, the next question they ask is usually "How do I know it will work for me? My body is different!" **I believe that we are all the same.** The Human Genome Project found that the two most diverse cultures or races on earth are more than 99.9 percent the same, genetically. The differences occur mostly in physical stature and traits that govern our appearance, such as the color of our eyes and texture of our hair. We all have a heart, lungs, brain, skin, stomach, skeleton, and all the rest that makes us human. When we are functioning as a healthy species, all our bodily functions are the same from person to person. The only differences are between the sexes (but we won't go there in this book).

What, then, makes us seem so different to one another? That would be our lifestyle—the way we live our lives. This is a spectrum of factors that includes how well we eat, our thinking patterns, whether we exercise, whether we believe in God or other Higher Power, the kind of work that we do, how we were raised as a child. These all have effects on our being, but probably the most important factor is stress and how we deal with it as an everyday component of living. It is this stress that weighs heavily on us (see the section earlier in this chapter). As I learned when working in the steel mill as a young man, even the strongest steel, when constantly stressed, will fatigue and break.

What is different from one person to another is only the type of stress each one experiences, and how they choose to deal with it. This creates unique symptoms in our bodies, though the underlying cause is always the same. Logically, then, if we use a process whereby we address the cause, all symptoms should disappear at some point. The ideal process consists of our cleansing and detoxifying the body, while at the same time we regenerate healthy tissues for it.

Good Side Effects

This process, like most, has side effects, but for a change they are good ones. They generally include less pain, increased energy, and a more positive outlook on life. All these benefits work to make it easier for us to be happy. When we become happy, we will heal faster and we will make good decisions that continue to foster this newborn sense of health and well-being.

I assure you that it is much easier to feel happy in a healthy body than in one wracked by pain or riddled with dis-ease. I know that you can choose differently, that you can make changes that will have long-lasting and positive effects on your whole life. With a healthy body, your mind will find peace and will start to open on a higher spiritual level, and other aspects of your life will continue to change and evolve as well. This can lead to a new-found sense of freedom and empowerment.

So now—at long last, and with high expectations—let's begin your Master Cleanse!

PART 2

Everything You Need to Know About the Master Cleanse

CHAPTER 6

The Master Cleanse

Resistance is futile! Give in to better health! It lies ahead for you, if you make yourself open to that prospect and finish reading this book.

You are now going to learn all the details about the amazing Master Cleanse. Specifically, you will read about how it will benefit you, how to prepare for it, what ingredients you need to obtain in advance, what to expect during the cleanse and after, how long to stay on it, how to come off it safely, and common mistakes that you will want to avoid.

Along the way, I will share with you a number of cases of clients and colleagues who experienced some truly astonishing results with the cleanse. (Also see the testimonials in Chapter 13.)

Benefits of the Cleanse

Over my many years of practice, people have reported myriad benefits that have come to them during or after doing a Master Cleanse. To give only the principal ones:

Better sleep—It is now more restful and deeper.

More energy—To the point where some people start following an exercise program, even though they had never before exercised in their entire life.

Clarity of mind—People tell me that a burst of awareness has come over them, almost frightening them, because after a cleanse they realize how out of touch they were with their bodies and their overall health.

Positive outlook—One woman called me on Day 37 to thank me for my help with her cleanse, because she no longer harbored thoughts of suicide.

Greater flexibility—Even yoga instructors who have done a cleanse have told me how astonished they were at their increased amount of physical flexibility.

Weight loss—Women often lose 1 pound per day during a cleanse, men up to 2 pounds.

Freedom from addictions—I have known many people who after a cleanse stop smoking, or using alcohol, or doing recreational drugs, or consuming junk foods, to name only a few.

Increased strength—During and after a cleanse, many people who like to work out can increase their weight load when at the gym, with all the side benefits that implies.

Swelling and pain—These conditions are often reduced.

Hair loss—People report their hair stops falling out and has more body.

Skin improves—Problem skin clears up, becomes healthier.

Allergies reduced—Some allergies are significantly lessened, and others can even disappear entirely after a cleanse or two.

You yourself may experience many more positive outcomes doing the Master Cleanse. This chapter will tell you all about how to do the cleanse.

First, mentally prepare yourself for the cleanse and all that it involves. Be aware that whenever people start a Master Cleanse on a whim, they also tend to go off it on a whim. It lacks importance to them, so no wonder they fail on it. Therefore, it's best to set a goal of at least 10 days on the Master Cleanse. Set those days aside and make sure you don't have a full calendar of social events. It usually is best not to tell too many people (or sometimes anyone outside your own home) that you are doing a cleanse.

Second, do not let others discourage you. I have seen many prospective cleanses aborted by third-party doubters and skeptics who have never themselves done the Master Cleanse or who, if they have done it, did it incorrectly. Sometimes such people have the nerve to speak authoritatively about it—as if you could learn how to swim by coaching others from the sidelines rather than plunging into the water yourself with a good instructor nearby. In your case, do not let others sabotage your efforts. You'll want to surround yourself with people who support you in your journey toward greater wellness.

How to Get Started

Some people like to prepare their body before a cleanse. They go on a vegetarian diet for four or five days before starting the cleanse, ramping up to an all-veggie diet before starting the cleanse itself. This simpler diet will be less stressful on the body and will help with the eventual elimination of some of your poor food choices. Eating such a diet will make it easier for you to transition to the Master Cleanse.

If you drink coffee or caffeinated soda every day, you will want to prevent the headaches that are caused by caffeine withdrawal. Start taking pantothenic acid (vitamin B-5) for about 4 days before starting the cleanse. The dosage should be approximately 400 mg., taken 3 times a day, while at the same time you reduce your coffee or soda intake about 25 percent each day. This will help you taper off the caffeine that you are accustomed to having. The day you start your cleanse, you will be off coffee or soda completely and will no longer need to take the vitamin supplement.

Most important, you will need to go out and gather your ingredients: lemons, maple syrup, cayenne pepper, herbal laxative, and sea salt. (See the sections below for full details, and the shopping list on page 66.) If you have no other source of good water, you will need to add bottled water to your list. Whenever possible, buy organic lemons to make your lemonade drink; it will taste much better and will also have a higher nutritional quality, not having been treated by pesticides, herbicides, and chemical fertilizers that are typically used in commercially grown produce. Some consumers might complain about the higher cost of organic produce, but remember that this is the only food you will be eating for 10 days or more—so get the best; you deserve it.

Contraindications and Cautions

People who have had organ transplants and are on immune-suppressant drugs *cannot* do the Master Cleanse. The cleanse will stimulate the immune system and also inhibit the effectiveness of the drugs, a combination that will likely cause the immune system to attack the transplanted organ and end in serious problems, if not worse. I believe, but I am not entirely sure, that most drugs are acid forming in the body. I do know that drugs should not be flushed down the toilet or thrown in the garbage, because they are considered to be toxic. Unused medication should be returned to the pharmacy.

Allergic to Lemons or Cayenne

The Master Cleanse uses lemons and cayenne, precisely because they possess properties good for stirring up toxicity in the body. Their effects, however, are often mislabeled or misunderstood. If you are already somewhat toxic and you are eating either lemon or cayenne, or both, and experiencing discomfort or what you think is an allergic reaction, this may be due to your body's attempting to cleanse itself *and* digest food at the same time. This creates a conflict; sometimes it even causes severe discomfort. When you are on the Master Cleanse you are not eating any other foods, so the issue of other food allergies does not arise.

Refer to Chapter 13, which contains a testimonial from an individual allergic to lemon or cayenne pepper.

Surrender to the Process

It can be hard to try something entirely new to your experience, especially if it's something that sounds a bit weird or even risky—even though you hear good things about it from people you trust.

You might try this little mental exercise that I often give to clients who are anxious. On first glance it seems odd, but it works:

1. *Know where you are.* Imagine that you have called a travel agent and are now asking her to book you a flight, but you have no idea where you are!

2. *Know where you are going.* Again call the travel agent and say, "I am in Seattle but I don't want to go to New York or Miami; not to Atlanta, either. I also don't like London as a destination." The agent, in frustration, will ask, "Well, where *do* you want to go?"

3. *Surrender to the process.* You know where you are and where you want to go. You now have to trust the travel agent, the airline, the taxi driver, the baggage handler, and all concerned that they will get you and your suitcase there. The agent will ask for the dates you want to travel and for payment. Your responsibility is only to show up at the airport at the right time on the proper day, and as if by magic you will soon arrive at your destination. You did not have to design the plane, build it, fuel it up, or fly it. *You just get on the plane!* You surrender to the process that others have established and tested.

Now apply this exercise to your current state of health and the goals you desire to achieve by using the Master Cleanse. Start by surveying your present state of health. Once you know where you are, move on to the next step—defining the results you want.

As you think about your first Master Cleanse, be flexible and open-minded about it, just as you would if you were flying overseas for the first time and felt a little anxious. In both situations, you could meet a little turbulence, or have to change flights partway there, or be bothered a bit by rough weather. Just trust yourself and be willing to roll with whatever comes up.

Don't get upset or disturbed if every little thing doesn't happen exactly the way you might have expected. This process can be exciting and adventurous. This journey toward better health may change your life, and will surely bring you much more that you might imagine.

It so happens that I am writing this paragraph on the exact day when, 27 years ago, I was taking a course on Stanley Burroughs's work. Did I know that that first step would start me on the long road to where I am today? No, but I did know it was absolutely the thing I wanted to do—so I surrendered myself to doing it with a happy heart.

How to Do the Master Cleanse

You must first read this book through to the end. Make notes or highlight steps or cautions or tips as you feel it helpful.

Make sure you understand how to do the Master Cleanse properly so that you can complete it with success and experience the results. I'm amused to recall that Stanley Burroughs would often say something that technical support people still tell their frustrated customers: "WAEFFTI—When All Else Fails, Follow The Instructions."

GOOD TO READ: IN THE MASTER'S VOICE

Some readers might profit from browsing through Stanley Burroughs's original volume, *Healing for the Age of Enlightenment*. The author self-published it in 1976; it was revised and reprinted in 1993. Though the book is sometimes out of print, a limited number of copies may be available through bookstores that can do online searches for used books, or through an Internet search engine or an online book vendor.

Follow these steps, in order (they are explained at length in the sections below).

1. Gather the ingredients.

2. Take an herbal laxative the night before you start the cleanse.

3. The next morning, repeat the laxative, or drink an internal salt water bath.

4. Be sure to have 3 or 4 bowel movements every day while using the laxative.

5. Now start to drink the lemonade, freshly made: 6 to 12 glasses each day.

I will explain each step in great detail, and over the course of the book I will repeat each instruction in various ways. You will not have to do any guessing or improvising.

Step 1 — Gather Ingredients

First, assemble all the ingredients you need to do your cleanse. Buy only enough lemons for about 3 days at a time if you can. If you wish to use limes instead of lemons, make sure that they are starting to be yellow in color, to be ripe; a dark green lime is unripe. A close friend did the Master Cleanse using only green, unripe limes and after several days complained that she felt sick with every glass of limeade she drank. Limes that have developed brown spots are now bitter tasting and should not be used.

It is best to keep lemons on a counter at room temperature, or even to set them in the sunlight; this allows them to ripen. I check my lemons and limes once or twice a day to make sure they are not starting to spoil. If they are ripening too quickly, I rub a small amount of lemon essential oil (see Chapter 9 and Resources section) on the lemon or lime peel to prevent spoilage.

Lemons and limes kept in the refrigerator will have a lower enzyme activity (which you don't want) and be less flavorful. If you have lemons refrigerated, if possible remove them about 2 days before you use them.

SHOPPING LIST

To prepare ingredients for a 10-day cleanse, you will need the following (approximately):
- 60 to 80 lemons (preferably organic)
- 2 quarts maple syrup
- ½ cup sea salt
- 10 gallons of good water (more if you want to drink it both as water and as tea)
- 2 ounces cayenne pepper
- Sufficient herbal laxative
- (If needed) set of measuring spoons, including ⅛ teaspoon size

TIP ON PURGING

Laxatives should always be used with caution. I have found that people who use herbal laxatives properly while on the Master Cleanse rarely have any negative effects. Laxatives should be used only for short periods of time while consuming food. Even herbal laxatives have side effects; some studies have shown serious side effects when senna, a substance commonly found in herbal laxatives, was taken in high dosages or for extended periods of time. Carefully read the ingredient list of any laxative you take, and restrict your usage of any laxative to only what is necessary. Seek professional advice regarding any long-term use of laxatives.

Step 2—Take an Herbal Laxative

With the ingredients all assembled, you will begin the Master Cleanse by taking an herbal laxative the night before you start. The laxative may be in the form of a tablet, capsule, or tea. If you prefer tea, make it according to instructions, but make a note of how strong it turns out; it may need to be steeped longer, or to have another tea bag added, to strengthen its effects. When using the laxative in tablet or capsule form, you generally need at least 3 to 5 of them to create the desired results. Whatever the form you take it in, the laxative must be used each and every night of the Master Cleanse. This will ensure that you eliminate all the toxins that your body is releasing.

The laxative may cause diarrhea symptoms in some people. If this occurs, stop taking it until the diarrhea has stopped. Please remember that this is a liquid monodiet, with no fiber whatsoever to bulk up in the colon. The continual ingestion of fluids, combined with the elimination of runny, slimy mucus and old waste, will make your bowel movements appear as though you have diarrhea. (In fact, you do not.) It can take 2 to 3 days for the stool to go from firm to rather loose. The diarrhea symptoms I am speaking of are manifested when you have to run repeatedly to the bathroom several times a day without much control of your colon.

Step 3—Repeat the Laxative, or Drink a Salt Water Bath

In the morning of Day 1 of the cleanse, before drinking lemonade, *either* repeat taking the herbal laxative *or* use an internal salt water bath. The internal salt water bath is made by adding **2 teaspoons** (not tablespoons) of uniodized sea salt to 1 quart of warm water. The salt water is mixed to the same salinity as your blood. When you drink this mixture, the salinity causes the water not to be absorbed into the bloodstream. You will not absorb the salt unless you are deficient in salt or the many trace minerals it contains. The salt water normally passes into the colon and out the rectum. You can drink the salt water bath every morning, or can omit it completely if you use the laxative instead. (I have taken the internal salt water bath hundreds of times, and I find it pleasant to do.)

There are several considerations to weigh before making your choice. The downside: The salt water bath can start to be eliminated within ½ hour, or can take up to 1½ hours to take effect after you drink it. The final elimination of the salt water will often come about 1 hour after your first elimination.

The upside to the salt water bath is that, with it, you will not have to make any urgent runs to the bathroom throughout the rest of the day. This is very helpful if, for example, you are in a dentist's chair with her hands in your mouth, or if you will be in a business meeting during the day or are traveling on an airplane (though you will try to avoid that). Occasionally someone will not pass the salt water on their initial attempts. If this happens, don't worry about it; just add more salt the next time.

The herbal laxative can cause cramping. This is usually the result of your colon's discharging some rather nasty stuff. At a certain point you will not want to overdo the laxative, because it may cause severe cramping, even nausea. I find that, for me, the laxative is better at eliminating waste from the colon, so I usually do the salt water bath only 3 times in a 10-day cleanse. I drink the salt water on Day 1, then again on Day 3 or 4, and finally on Day 7 or 8.

Please do *not* drink the quart of salt water all at one time, as you will probably throw it up and be disgusted with it. I take about 10 minutes to drink my salt water, and I warm it to body temperature before consuming it. Some people imagine they are drinking a salty soup or broth, which seems to work for them. You may find the salt water distasteful at first, but after a short time you can get used to it and it will become easy to swallow.

Step 4 — Have Daily Bowel Movements

It is vital that you have at least 3 to 4 eliminations from your bowel each day when you are using the herbal laxative. Some people experience what they colorfully describe as a "Ring of Fire" during elimination. To be plain about it, this is merely a combination of the cayenne pepper and acidic waste being passed from the bowel. The best remedy is usually to apply coconut oil on the affected area. Do not use hand cream or lotion on tender tissues, as they usually contain severely irritating chemicals.

Step 5 — Start Drinking the Lemonade

The first morning of the cleanse and every morning thereafter, you begin to drink the lemonade when you are hungry (normally within the first hour or two after arising), or, if doing the salt water bath, drink the lemonade after you begin eliminating the salt water. Drink 6 to 12 glasses of lemonade every day. Drink the lemonade whenever you are hungry, and try not to let yourself get overly hungry. Remember that while the Master Cleanse is a simple process, many people create a little difficulty with it. Therefore, please follow instructions carefully.

Mix Your Lemonade

Place 2 tablespoons of freshly squeezed lemon juice into a glass.

Add 2 tablespoons of maple syrup (use a measuring spoon for accuracy).

Add 1/10 teaspoon of cayenne powder.

Fill the glass with 8 ounces of good-quality water.

Stir and drink up!

TIP ON JUICING

Treat yourself to a good-quality electric citrus juicer. Juicers of that type are far more efficient than hand juicers and will produce more juice than if you squeeze by hand or utensil.

Always drink your lemonade fresh. Drink it within 10 minutes after you prepare it. Drink it whenever you feel hungry. Start drinking the lemonade about 1 hour after taking your laxative, or after your first elimination of the salt water bath. Drink 6 to 12 glasses a day (each mixture amounting to at least 10 fluid ounces). I suggest that, unless you are obese, you consume at least 8 glasses of the lemonade mixture each day. I myself often drink 12 glasses a day, and will drink as many as 16 glasses if I am extremely physically active. I have known someone to drink 24 to 26 glasses a day (that is, 2 gallons!) while training for a triathlon, and to do so for 12 days in a row.

If you feel hungry, tired, or cold, it is often because you are not drinking enough lemonade. If the lemonade tastes too sweet or you want to lose weight, you can decrease the maple syrup in each drink by 1 tablespoon. If you desire to maintain or gain weight, however, you may add 1 tablespoon maple syrup to each drink.

OPTION: For those people who cannot make their lemonade fresh for each drink—because they will be away from home—there is a simple alternative. Mix equal parts of maple syrup and lemon juice as a concentrate into a dark container and keep it cool, if possible; a thermos is ideal. Prepare enough concentrate to last as long as you will be away. Whenever you hanker for a glass of lemonade, measure 4 tablespoons of this concentrate into a glass, add the cayenne pepper and the water, stir, and drink. The maple syrup will act as a preservative for the lemon juice, which in turn will help to prevent oxidation of the vitamin C and the enzymes. Note that as soon as you add water you must drink it—say, within 5 to 10 minutes.

You can alternate drinking water or herbal tea throughout the day with the lemonade. It is important, however, not to drink too much water and not enough lemonade. Drink water or herbal tea if you feel dehydrated or when the weather is hot. Remember, you must drink at least 6 glasses of lemonade per day!

Never microwave your lemonade. Doing so will destroy many of its valuable enzymes and vitamins and will diminish its effectiveness.

Follow these simple steps—to the letter!—and you will be most likely to succeed by having a good, productive Master Cleanse.

Master Cleanse Ingredients and Their Properties

You might be wondering, "Where will I get the energy I need during the cleanse, if I eat nothing at all?"

Maple Syrup

The ingredient in the Master Cleanse program that provides you with the fuel for your body over the period of the cleanse is pure maple syrup—plain and simple. Stanley Burroughs recommended it because of its high quality as a food as well as its general availability. You may use raw cane syrup or freshly pressed cane juice, if available, instead of maple syrup.

Maple syrup's properties are what make it suitable for a cleanse. Maple syrup contains a number of minerals and vitamins, in trace amounts. Depending on where the syrup was collected, the amount of nutrients varies, as does the taste. Both are determined by mineral content in the soil and the growing conditions of the maple trees. Potassium, calcium, magnesium, manganese, phosphorus, sodium, iron, zinc, copper, tin, sulfur, and silicon can be found in maple syrup. Vitamins A, B-1, B-2, B-5, B-6, biotin, and folic acid are present as well, along with a minuscule amount of amino acids.

Maple syrup is generally marketed in four grades. Some confusion can arise between the old and the current grading system. The old system had A, B, and C grades. The current grading system runs from lightest to darkest: Gr. [Grade] A Light Amber, Gr. A Medium Amber, Gr. A Dark Amber, and finally Gr. B. The problem began with the original system, where Gr. A was considered better than Gr. B and, of course, much better than Gr. C, which led to large differences between the A and B grades in selling price. At one time I have seen Gr. A sell for twice the price of Gr. C, although now all grades sell at roughly the same price. Canadians will need to use #2 Amber grade.

The difference in the grades is a result of the time period in which the sap is collected from the maple trees in the spring. The first run of sap is called Gr. A Light Amber. This consists of sap that the maple tree stores in its roots over the winter. The warm days and cold nights make the sap run up into the tree, and will act as an antifreeze and also feed the tree. The reserves in the roots, as they are used up, urge the roots to now absorb moisture from the soil and to continue to pump sap up into the tree. This new uptake of water by the roots brings with it trace minerals from the soil that will darken the sap.

This first run, Gr. A Light Amber, is light in both color and taste, owing to its lack of minerals. During the winter the sap in the roots loses some of its mineral content. The Gr. A Medium Amber is a combination of older, light sap mixed with newer and heavier sap laden with minerals. As the season progresses, the concentration of minerals continues to increase and Gr. A Dark Amber is the next run. The final run of sap, or Gr. B, is all new uptake from the roots and has the highest mineral content.

Gr. B maple syrup is actually the highest quality syrup for the Master Cleanse, and the best possible choice. Stanley recommended Gr. B (or what was called Gr. C); if neither is available, get the darkest grade you can buy. One tablespoon of maple syrup supplies about 55 calories (or 220 per quarter cup, which is equivalent to 4 tablespoons).

Other Sugars or Sweeteners You must never substitute any artificial sweetener, such as Splenda, Equal, aspartame, or honey (which has been predigested by the bee). Honey is created from nectar and natural sugar.

Agave is another sweetener that is becoming widely available, though it is not a good choice for the Master Cleanse. It is made from the agave plant, which is high in a compound called inulin (or fructosan), which is extracted as a dark juice, filtered to remove minerals, and heated to convert the inulin into fructose. Finally, it is concentrated to make syrup. Usually two grades of agave juice are available—light and dark.

GOOD TO KNOW

Inulin is an indigestible carbohydrate that is completely soluble. Since it is a natural fiber, it can be mixed into any type of food or liquid without affecting the taste. It comes in a powder form and dissolves. The most common source of inulin is chicory root. Inulin is a prebiotic—that is, it stimulates the growth of beneficial bacteria that live naturally in the colon.

Fructose is a sugar used extensively by the processed food industry and soda drink manufacturers. It has been made widely available from the production of corn syrup. Fructose has a low glycemic index. This lowered insulin secretion fools the body into not recognizing the caloric intake; this, in turn, blocks the body's ability to regulate food intake or to control weight gain. This missing "feedback loop" makes you consume more foods, which are then converted to...you guessed it, fat.

Any sugar that is good for your health should be produced by a single-stream method of manufacture. This means one product in and only one product out—not multistream, which results in the removal of various amounts of mineral content. This is an extremely

Sugary Treats...for Kids?!

Two decades ago, when foods' effects were far less known than they are today, my two young children attended a fine arts preschool set up by parents. I expressed some concern about the quality of some foods that various parents brought to the school for snack time, on a rotating basis. We all eventually agreed that candy or foods with white sugar would not be allowed, and instead that the preferred snack would be raw fruits and vegetables. I often chatted with the young instructors while waiting for my children to get ready to leave. These young women would politely listen to my mini-lectures on the importance of eating unprocessed foods and cleansing regularly. One day when I came to pick up my kids from school, all four instructors rushed over to me, anxious to tell me something. That day, one child had brought cupcakes with sugar icing to celebrate her birthday with her schoolfriends. The instructors thought they could bend the rules and let the children eat the sugary treats. When they did so, they soon found the children becoming hyperactive and unmanageable from the sudden surge of sugar into their bloodstream. The teachers lost control of them, so they had the children go into the gym to run off their energy spike. *Moral of the story*: Many nutritionists and health practitioners today call processed sugar a drug—because it rapidly changes mood and alters body chemistry in undesirable ways.

important point, because it is whole sugars' natural mineral content that makes them safe for consumption. (Maple syrup that is 100 percent syrup is "whole," or unadulterated, and therefore safe.)

I have known of a practitioner who restricts his clients' use of agave to only 10 days of the cleanse. People doing more than that were found to be suffering from demineralization. It's logical that eating demineralized foods (that is, all processed or whitened foods) causes the body to go into "mineral debt." This results in specific organs being weakened by the lack of proper nutrients, making them unable to function properly or to replicate their cells normally.

If you ever read pirate-and-treasure stories as a youth, you may have heard about the crew that was shipwrecked in the Bahamas while carrying a precious cargo of sugar from Caribbean planta-tions to the Old World (Europe). A storm forced their ship onto a reef, where it foundered and was about to go down. Some of the crew swam to shore, and were able to salvage portions of the cargo. The members of the crew who ate the processed sugar for several days were said to have gone quite crazy, while those who consumed only food scavenged from the island stayed well until they were rescued. Lesson learned?

Glucose and the Pancreas   Your body burns glucose, and only glucose, for fuel. *Everything* that you metabolize as energy comes from glucose created from carbohydrates, proteins, or fats. Many people have found themselves to be highly sensitive to sugar from their overconsumption of processed sugars and starches since childhood. This acquired sensitivity can cause them to experience both high and low fluctuations of energy. The sufferers often compensate for these unpleasant feelings by eating even *more* complex carbohydrates, proteins, and some fats, thus worsening the cycle.

Complex carbohydrates have a lower glycemic index and raise blood sugars more slowly than do simple sugars, such as pastries or other baked goods using white flour and white sugar. Proteins and fats have to be converted by the liver into sugar; this requires a longer lead time to release sugar into the body, and makes for its more-regular influx into the bloodstream. This slower and more-regular uptake of fuel by the body enables the pancreas to keep blood sugar levels properly balanced. The problem with this approach is that it is only symptomatic, not causative. My analogy for this: If you accidentally knocked a hole into a wall of your house, would you hang a nice picture over it—or would you repair it?

As you can probably imagine, the new dietary lifestyle that many people follow these days, including eating more complex carbohydrates, is actually only a mask. People think they're doing the right thing, eating the right foods, which indeed they are, on one level. But they have not addressed the root cause. I have seen these people eat fruit and still experience the roller-coaster ride of imbalanced sugar levels. Take the picture down off the wall 10 years later, and the hole is still there. We should fix the problem at its source, not just give it (so to speak) a "sugar coating." Recent research has found that the HIV virus, which causes AIDS, is sugar coated, allowing it to hide from the immune system and be readily absorbed by the cell.

When a pancreas suffers damage by excessive processed foods and white sugar, it also suffers nutritional deficiencies from the lack of many minerals and vitamins. One job of that organ is to regulate blood sugar levels to within 1/10th of 1 percent. It now should be obvious to you that devitalized foods and foods devoid of minerals and vitamins do a double whammy on the pancreas: Their lack of nutrients weaken it, and the dramatic rise in blood sugar levels from the easy absorption of these foods stresses that organ by pushing it to overproduce insulin. This causes the roller-coaster high and lows that many people experience throughout the day, even though they think they're eating "normally."

This rocky ride often stems from childhood. How frequently do you "reward" your own children with a sugar-laced treat or candy, or see other parents do so? The child receiving this reward starts to associate love and care with sugar, at an unconscious level, and thus learns to crave it in order to feel good. Why do you think we call certain foods "comfort food"? We have made an error of associating certain kinds of foods with love and attention. Just try to watch television while doing the Master Cleanse, and you will be surprised at the food commercials and how they will make you tempted to eat. (I have not consumed burgers for decades and normally I am not interested in eating them, but when I am on the cleanse and I see TV ads showing juicy burgers I sure do want to eat one.)

Stevia   A sweetener that many people ask about using on the Master Cleanse is Stevia, also known as sweetleaf or sugarleaf. This product is not a true sugar but a compound extracted from a very sweet but indigestible herb in the sunflower family. It provides no calories or energy at all while on the cleanse. Therefore, if you use it you will be starving yourself—something you do not want to do.

Lemons

A unique food, the lemon is in a class all its own. (A lime is chemically equivalent.) Lemon is an acid food—yet, paradoxically, it is highly alkalizing to the body when digested. The several acids in lemon help to break down various calcified substances throughout the body, such as kidney stones and gallstones. The high levels of potassium, calcium, and magnesium found in a lemon makes it an optimal choice to alkalize the body's tissues.

You likely have smelled lemon essence in many cleaning agents, polishes, and soaps. Lemon juice is used extensively to clean computer chips in the high-tech industry. Lemon is also a natural cleansing agent for the body's insides, as it breaks and loosens mucus to be eliminated. This property has made it a common home remedy for treating colds and flulike symptoms. For example, whenever I feel the rare cold coming on, I drink a glass of lemonade with plenty of cayenne pepper, and usually all my symptoms disappear within an hour or two.

A lemon contains calcium, magnesium, potassium, phosphorus, sodium, zinc, copper, selenium, and iron—but there's even more to it than that. Lemon is the only fruit or vegetable that contains more anions than cations. *Anions* are atoms or molecules that carry a negative charge, while *cations* are atoms or molecules that carry a positive charge. This positive (or negative) charge will determine a food's properties when consumed by the body. This anionic quality is much the same as in saliva, bile, the stomach's digestive fluids, and digestive enzymes. All of these assist the body in autolysis (or self-digestion, as described in Chapter 5), in which it breaks down unhealthy tissues and cells that it then recycles to regenerate itself.

Lemons are high in vitamin C, as you no doubt know. They also contain lesser amounts of thiamine, riboflavin, niacin, pantothenic acid (vitamin B-5), and vitamin B-6. In addition, they contain a small amount of protein and fiber, plus an assortment of other trace nutrients. There are about 4 insignificant calories per tablespoon of lemon.

Do *not* use Meyer lemons for the Master Cleanse. While these are delicious in baked goods, they are unsuitable for the cleanse because they are less acidic and have slightly different properties.

Meyer lemons are considered a cross between a true lemon and a mandarin orange; in southern Texas they are called Valley lemons.

Cayenne Pepper

Herbologists often refer to cayenne as the Master Herb. It is typically ground from the pods and seeds of pungent, long, tapering red peppers of the genus *Capsicum*. When mixed with most other herbs in combination, cayenne acts as a catalyst—that is, it makes the other herbs react, and thus work more effectively. Cayenne pepper is a stimulant that raises metabolism, increases circulation by purifying and thinning the blood, and helps many digestive disorders. You might be amazed to learn that, when placed under the tongue as a tincture or powder, cayenne can even stop a heart attack. It will halt internal bleeding, and it can even be applied directly as first aid to external areas of the body that are bleeding.

Like lemon, cayenne breaks up and loosens mucus in the body. This benefits the sinuses, the bronchial tubes, and the lungs and allows clearer and easier breathing. Cayenne is high in both vitamins A and C, and contains some B vitamins as well. It also contains potassium and calcium, both of which make it highly alkalizing to the body. Capsaicin is the most active compound found in cayenne. It is cayenne's *heat* that we sense by both taste and touch (which is why Asian and Mexican chefs wear rubber gloves when handling certain superhot chili peppers). Its heat is what makes cayenne a pain reliever to the body; it is an ingredient in numerous over-the-counter products and ointments.

Cutting Corners

One day, while working in my garage cutting wood with a table saw, I got careless for a moment and put my index finger into the blade. It caused a deep injury, but did not cut to the bone, and it bled profusely. I dashed into my kitchen, opened the cayenne pepper container, and poured cayenne directly onto the injury. In about 5 to 10 seconds the cayenne pepper formed a barrier that stopped the bleeding entirely. It did sting for a minute or two, but after I stopped swearing I was happy to see the bleeding stop. My finger is fine today, but I still bear a scar that reminds me of that moment when cayenne saved the day.

A pepper's hotness is measured in Scoville units; cayenne typically ranges from 40,000 to 100,000 on this scale. I suggest that people unfamiliar with cayenne start at the bottom end of the scale. When cayenne pepper is not rated by the packager, it is generally at the 40,000 Scoville units level. Always test the hotness of the cayenne by using a small amount until you become familiar with its properties and how it affects your system.

You can purchase cayenne in most supermarkets, usually in the spice section, as well as at organic food stores and health food stores. Purchase cayenne pepper that is deep red or orange. Cayenne fades in color with age and should be stored in a cool, dark place.

TIP

To measure cayenne for the lemonade: Use a measuring spoon set. The smallest spoon in the set is usually 1/8 teaspoon; fill it about three-quarters full. Many people find the cayenne hot at first, so you may want to begin with less than 1/10 of a teaspoon and work up to the full amount.

Water

In addition to maple syrup, lemon, and cayenne, water is the final vital component of the Master Cleanse. As fetuses, we spent most of our first nine months suspended in amniotic fluid in the womb; that fluid is mostly water. Our body consists of about 70 percent water, so the need for good water for proper health cannot be overstressed. Water is the universal solvent and is likely needed universally to support life (one reason that scientists are always trying to find water on other planets or moons). It will dissolve more compounds than any other fluid.

This is an important point, because by now you know that the cleanse is designed first to break up, loosen, and dissolve wastes and toxins in the body and then to flush them out. You probably know that your body uses water to help flush and transport toxins to the organs of elimination (the colon, bladder, lungs, skin, and so on) to discharge them. Some people believe that many health problems can be significantly improved, or completely eliminated, with just an adequate consumption of good water.

I cannot overstate the importance of using good water during the Master Cleanse. Depending on the source and treatment of your city's water supply, you may have excellent water coming directly out of your tap. A vast number of brands of bottled water can be purchased today in stores and supermarkets, or can be home-delivered; I cannot comment on them or recommend one over another. A few cities still maintain artesian wells as free-flowing sources of good water. Water treatment systems in the home are growing in popularity because of some cities' or counties' questionable quality of tap water. Avoid chlorinated and fluoridated water.

In your cleanse, try to use water that is free of impurities or chemicals added by water treatment facilities. An often overlooked but important quality is water's pH level (its acidity or alkalinity, on a scale that ranges from 0 to 14; "pH" stands for "potential of hydrogen"). The Master Cleanse is designed to alkalize your body, so it is most important that you learn the pH level of the water source you will be using. Water for cleansing or drinking is best when the pH level is 7.0 or slightly higher. You can buy an inexpensive water pH testing kit (available at most drugstores) to help you determine what water is best for you to drink; Abundant Health is one among many distributors of pH strips (at a cost of about two cents per strip).

In addition to the Master Cleanse program, some people choose to do a water fast. They take in only water for several days, or even weeks. Stanley Burroughs, developer of the Master Cleanser, did not believe that people should do a water fast unless they first did the cleansing. When I was practicing in Toronto I treated several individuals who did water fasting regularly before they came to me for treatment. These people said they felt better, had more energy, and had significantly better results from the

Master Cleanse. I have never water fasted myself, so I cannot make a qualified judgment on the pros and cons of this therapy.

Reverse Osmosis Water   Water that is put through reverse osmosis (called RO water) is sometimes used for a Master Cleanse, though it is not ideal for that purpose. Such water goes through a dual filtration system: First it is filtered through carbon and then through a thin membrane that allows some water to flow through while catching and rejecting most impurities. This system has one major drawback, in addition to cost: About 75 percent of the water is rejected and is dumped down the drain, thereby wasting it. Acidifying the water before it comes to the membrane will make the filter more efficient, thus wasting less water and producing more filtered water. Such acidified water is detrimental to the Master Cleanse and is best *not* to be used.

Distilled Water   Stanley did not recommend using distilled water; he colorfully, if truthfully, said it was "cooked." The distillation process boils off oxygen as it is dissolved and removes many useful trace minerals that are naturally found in the water. Distilled water is also slightly acidic. If you need to use distilled water, I suggest that you set covered containers of it outside in the sun for 2 or 3 days to be recharged and then add back trace minerals by shaking a few grains of sea salt into it or by adding a few drops of a trace mineral supplement in liquid form.

My Own Water Preferences   I myself use a water ionizer, both for my drinking water and for doing the Master Cleanse. This unit has a carbon filtration system and uses a process that creates two streams of water—one acid, one alkaline. The alkalinity of the resulting water can be adjusted from about pH 7.0 to 9.0, depending on the acidity of your tap water. Many other treatment systems are available. I have even heard of some good systems that use magnets, though I cannot speak to their efficacy.

I have developed a rather unusual technique to enhance not only the taste but also the quality of the water I drink and use for the Master Cleanse. Suspend your disbelief here, please! I store my water in a glass, one-gallon, covered container that bears the labels **GRATITUDE** and **LOVE**. This may sound strange indeed, but the water simply tastes better after being in a container with those two words.

Masaru Emoto, a scientist and researcher in Japan, has made famous the way in which water can be imprinted by being exposed to music, pictures, or words. His book *The Hidden Messages in Water* shows numerous photographs and examples of how water that is frozen into tiny ice crystals is affected by its environment. He discovered this quite by accident. He first exposed liquid water to a specific piece of music, then froze some droplets (to make ice crystals) and proceeded to photograph them. He found that certain music made beautiful crystals, while other music—such as heavy metal—created malformed ones. He went on to expose water to words and phrases. I believe doing so would have an effect similar to exposing water to music. Positive or uplifting words had a marked effect on enhancing the beauty of the crystals. Negative words did the opposite. This has many implications. You might think this outlandish, but science is always exploring new frontiers.

Abundant Health, a distributor of pH strips for testing water, also sells stick-on, reusable labels that bear a variety of positive words. You can place labels of your choice on your water containers to charge them with the feeling or thought. (See the Resources section.)

The principles of homeopathy are consistent with this water-imprinting work. A homeopathic remedy is made by diluting a medicine in an aqueous solution to such a degree that the original compound is virtually undetectable. This extreme dilution still carries the signature of the concentrated compound in the water. For centuries people throughout the world have used homeopathy. It is becoming increasingly popular as an alternative holistic therapy, because some people experience great success with it.

Use of Supplements You should *not* use supplements while on the Master Cleanse. Such nutrients (whether in pill or liquid form) will stimulate your digestive processes and may even stop the detoxification process—something you do not want to happen. The Master Cleanse works effectively, as I have detailed it.

A few supplements are known to not interfere with the cleansing process and, in fact, to assist the body in healing. Herbs and herbal teas of all types (but without adding anything, such as honey or other sweetener) can be used with the cleanse. I strongly recommend the use of parasitic remedies (see Chapter 11). Digestive enzymes may be used while on the Master Cleanse, since they are not a food. These enzymes will assist the lemon and cayenne to break down undigested food and waste that have built up in the colon. I have taken as many as 10 enzyme capsules at a time, 3 or 4 times a day, while on the cleanse, and have noticed an increase in the number and bulk of my eliminations. As always, it is important to use good-quality enzymes; these can be obtained through a number of resources, including most health food stores and many online sites.

Essential Oils It is acceptable to ingest essential oils for the cleanse, as they do not need to be digested and are already in their simplest form to be used by the body. I take certain essential oils by mouth while on the cleanse. Drops of lemon essential oil can be added to your lemonade, and essential oils can be encapsulated and taken internally. **DO NOT** ingest essential oils, however, unless you absolutely know that they are therapeutic grade. There is more information to be found on this topic in Chapter 9.

What to Expect During the Master Cleanse

You need to know some of the ups as well as the downs of the Master Cleanse, because you will respond differently to the detoxification process than the next person. While I myself have only had positive experiences with the Master Cleanse, and while I know many people who have had successes similar to mine, a few folks will become troubled by physical or emotional issues that arise during their cleanse.

Over many years of practice and consulting, I have learned that everyone has his or her own unique experience with their first cleanse. I also know that each successive cleanse can be quite different from the first one. About 4 in 10 people may experience headaches, joint pain, low energy, and a general feeling of malaise at one or more stages during the cleanse. This is not at all unusual, because your body is going through withdrawal from sugar, caffeine, and other addictive foods, while at the same time familiarizing itself with a low-protein liquid diet, *and* at the same time stirring up toxic wastes in your body that will be eliminated. These symptoms are, in fact, caused not by the Master Cleanse but by what you have done to your body in the past.

Flashbacks of Feelings or Tastes

The Master Cleanse is something like a time machine, in that it takes you back in time and you reexperience old symptoms or conditions as you stir up the old toxins in your body. These old toxins are stored because of stress. In the same way, the Master Cleanse can free the same emotions and feelings that were left unfinished in some way.

I have had people on the Master Cleanse say they can taste cigarettes in their mouth, yet they have not smoked for many years. People who did recreational drugs years ago sometimes feel high, or "stoned," as old drugs get released from fat cells in the body. I have witnessed people get dilated pupils as they cleanse. One client had done chemotherapy recently and indicated that he was still burping the drugs up after 27 days of being on the cleanse. People will speak of craving foods they have not eaten for 10 years or so; the toxins from these foods are now entering the bloodstream and triggering old memories.

In the past, I typically had my clients come in for a consultation and then come back to have a Vita-Flex treatment during the period that they were on the cleanse. (See Chapter 7 for complete details of this adjunctive therapy.) During the Vita-Flex treatment, certain points on the feet would be supersensitive to my touch, indicating that a specific area of the body was experiencing a lack of wellness. I would ask if they now have, or have had, a problem in that specific area; sometimes my clients would say, "No, no problems there." About Day 5 or 6 they would call me and tell me that yes, they are having a problem, and "Guess where?" I would patiently explain to them that I could tell there was indeed a problem, but it had not yet surfaced. (Remember that dis-ease starts in the mind and manifests itself in the body.) I would add, maybe a bit smugly, that they were lucky to have caught it before it became a major problem. And together we would tackle the problem and come up with a solution.

You cannot always know what to expect, even when it seems obvious or logical to you. I have treated people who had been given only a week to live, yet after they started the Master Cleanse they would immediately begin feeling better. I also had a friend who once described himself as "healthy as a horse," though he could not last even one day on the Master Cleanse. Several months later this friend confided in me that his usual regimen, before doing the cleanse, included eating five or six chocolate bars each day, apparently without its affecting his health! He seemed oblivious to the amount of caffeine and white sugar he was regularly ingesting—but he felt the consequences when he began the Master Cleanse and couldn't stay on it.

Healing Crisis: A Good Thing

The 4 out of 10 people who do the cleanse and have a little trouble with it usually say they have one day in particular that is hardest to get through. They explain that it is not always a physical condition or discomfort that they are feeling. People who facilitate or work with others doing detoxification programs of one sort or another often describe such symptoms as a "healing crisis."

Crises of this type occur when the various organs of elimination are forced to function at an accelerated pace, in order to deal with a sudden influx of wastes from the various tissues in the body. (Think of a flash flood rushing down a bone-dry riverbed.) The symptoms can be really dramatic, but may only last minutes; in some people, they can last several hours or more.

When people I have treated call me to say they are dying, I calmly reply, "No, you're not dying. You are getting better." They protest that idea and again say, "Really, I'm dying!" Of course, I can detect from their intonation that they are just feeling bad, so I assure them that what's happening is that they are getting better—but feeling worse for the moment. These bad feelings often clear up after the person has eliminated. If it continues for more than a day, I suggest to them that they consider doing one or more of Stanley Burroughs's adjunctive therapies, such as Vita-Flex and Color Therapy. (See Chapters 7 and 8.) After using these therapies some people can, in only minutes, completely alleviate all or most symptoms.

A healing crisis is actually beneficial, though it is often misinterpreted by people and may be the very thing that causes them to halt the cleansing process. Psychotherapists sometimes explain to their patients the distinction between having a mental "breakdown" and experiencing a "breakthrough" in self-awareness and understanding. The same holds true with the physical body.

Menstrual Cycle Changes or Blood Donation

Many women to whom I have recommended the Master Cleanse report that while on the cleanse their menstrual cycle started at a different time of the month than usual. This is a typical reaction. They go on to say that their discharges are often darker and heavier, but only temporarily. I assure them that they need not be concerned about the blood loss on the Master Cleanse. I have even had clients donate blood while on the cleanse, which has greatly surprised me. (Most people would never consider doing such a thing while on a cleanse.)

Comfort Food

Many people eat comfort food, discussed earlier, which is the consuming of something (usually something unhealthy) to displace emotional discomfort. When the coping mechanism is taken away (that is, they run out of that yummy food or that heavenly drink or that pep-up snack), they feel distressed. But drinking lemonade on the Master Cleanse does not act like your favorite comfort food, nor will it ever replace it. Now, wait: This is not a bad thing. In fact, it creates an opportunity for you to deal with some past experience in a real way so that you can let it go.

I have seen people become angry, sad, or confused during the cleanse, as the detoxification process stirs up their feelings. I reas-

---

Mind Helps Body Help Mind

On a trip I met a shy young woman. After talking with her I advised her to read the Burroughs book and try a Master Cleanse. Later, she called me on Day 3 to say she was feeling great and had lots of energy. On Day 7 she phoned to tell me that she had low energy, hated how the drink tasted, and wanted to stop. I replied that stopping the cleanse when you're feeling bad is not the best thing to do and assured her that she was going through a healing crisis: her physical symptoms were an expression of a deeper underlying emotion.

We spoke for quite a while. Remembering my first impression of how she looked uncomfortable with her appearance, I drew her out about it, asking her what had happened in the past to cause her to shut down. She got quiet, and eventually told me of an incident when she was about 5 years old and her grandmother caught her innocently admiring herself in a mirror and thinking how beautiful she looked. She was scolded and shamed for this, and as a result had stopped loving her physical being. She felt the effects to the present day. I suggested that she forgive her grandmother (who had since died), start to love herself fully as a woman, and let her beauty and femininity express itself freely. (I went into more detail with these suggestions.) She stayed on the cleanse, and called me on Day 10 to say that all her energy was back, that she felt very happy, and even that the lemonade drink tasted great and was totally satisfying her needs. Again, *mind helps body help mind*.

---

sure them that these feelings are like clouds; they will pass, and the sun will shine again. Doing a Master Cleanse can make clear what our emotional relationships with food really are.

Other Conditions During a Cleanse

It is rare but not uncommon to feel *nausea* during the cleanse. The queasy feeling usually disappears after the individual throws up. Most people report that what they vomit up is only mucus and that they feel fine afterward. I have known only three or four people whose nausea did not dissipate, even when they tried drinking ginger tea. If the problem persists for more than one day, I suggest that the person stop the cleanse and attempt it again in a week or so. The wait is often all that is needed for the cleanse to work.

You can also expect to have *bad breath,* since you are breathing out toxins from your lungs and your mouth. *Body odor* also becomes worse, because you are excreting toxins through your skin. Your *bowel movements* can smell terribly foul. All of these are not a bad thing—they are better coming out than staying in and continuing to poison your body.

You may also feel your *sinuses* draining and *mucus* loosening in your throat. Your *skin* may worsen for a short time as well. All are indications that these organs have been overloaded in the past and are now letting go of various irritants. Such conditions generally do not last long and are not troubling.

During the cleanse, it is important that you assess your own experience with it and decide whether you wish to continue giving it your very best try. If you experience a *healing crisis* during your cleanse, as described above, you will have to make a judgment as to what to do. At that point you might seek support, use supportive therapies, or stop the cleanse and consider trying again at a later date when you feel stronger or more hopeful. (See Resources for some guidance on support.)

Having Problems During the Cleanse?

As I say several times throughout this book, the Master Cleanse is obviously not a program for everyone. But it isn't always easy to tell in advance whether a given person will take to the cleanse, tolerate it, and end up benefiting from it.

I have known many clients and even friends to endure tremendous discomfort and pain on a cleanse, to a degree that I myself would probably not want to put up with. Yet most were highly motivated people who were willing to experience a healing crisis to get to the other side and feel well. For most people the worst day is usually Day 3 of the cleanse. Other common problem days are Days 1 and 4. Having a problem day occurs about 40 percent of the time, but the number of problems experienced skyrockets if the cleanse is done incorrectly. The most common mistakes are: not drinking the lemonade fresh, omitting the laxative, and not drinking adequate amounts of lemonade. Almost daily I talk to someone on the cleanse who is experiencing problems, and a large percentage of these people are doing it wrong—wrong ingredients, wrong amounts, wrong timing, wrong foods before the cleanse.

My own experience was—and continues to be—very positive and enjoyable. During the time that I was writing this book, I did the Master Cleanse three times. In all my years of experience, I have never had any healing crises, headaches, or pains while on the cleanse. No, wait a minute...I spoke too soon: I do remember that, during my fourth cleanse, I started to get canker sores. This is not at all unusual, as the cleanse is also correcting the tissues in the mouth. After two or three days of sores, someone from my Stanley Burroughs training suggested using a recommendation of his: gargling with a half and half mixture of apple cider vinegar and water several times a day. That was all I had to do, and my canker sores completely cleared up.

I attribute my continued success with the cleanse to my maintaining a positive attitude about the cleanse and having a clear expectation of its benefits. I tell myself that I deserve to have a good result, and I always get one. Conversely, I have seen people embark on the cleanse with a lot of fear and trepidation, experience some discomfort that they interpret as a problem (and a failure of the Master Cleanse *for them*), and so they stop immediately.

> **Date-Death by Pizza**
>
> A friend was doing the Master Cleanse. By Day 10 she had lost about a dozen pounds and was looking so good that men started approaching her for dates. She was not prepared for such a dramatic change and found it hard to deal with all this new attention. But guess what? She chose to come off the cleanse by eating...drum-roll here...*pizza!* To no one's surprise, she gained back all her weight, and the attention went away. Self-defeatingly, she had set and met her own limitations.

Some people expect the worse and in fact feel worse, in a kind of self-fulfilling prophecy. Yet some of these same people, while doing medical interventions, lose their hair, or get extremely weak, or live in constant pain, or have diarrhea and many more side effects, and still are willing to endure the treatment without question because they trust the authority who recommended it.

Permitting Yourself to Heal

One of the biggest stumbling blocks is for people to "Argue for your own limitations." This is the height of self-defeating expectations! I have personally heard hundreds, probably thousands, of reasons why the Master Cleanse can't work for someone. People will insist to me that "My condition is special!" I start laughing at such people and ask them: "Why would God, or your Higher Power, or Evolution, or Intelligent Design bless *you* with a condition or problem that cannot be solved or healed?" My advice? Get out of your own way. Allow yourself to heal, and then accept it as a gift!

The mind will play tricks on us whenever our intention is not clearly stated or firmly in mind when we take up new endeavors. A study was done to see whether luck was a measurable factor in people's lives. The researchers found that the people who believed in luck had more of it than people who did not believe in luck.

Applying this information to the Master Cleanse, or to anything else in your life for that matter—whether it be a new job, a challenging adventure, or a promising relationship—clearly requires that you follow one principle: "To experience the best, we must expect the best."

Weight Loss

It is not unusual for men to lose up to 2 pounds a day while on the Master Cleanse. For women, alas, the loss is a little slower. Women tend to lose about 1 pound a day, but can go as high as 1½ pounds a day. Remember, it is not only fat that is burning off. Excess fluids, old waste, and unhealthy tissues are also being dumped, like the junk going up the conveyor belt at a recycling center. Once you meet your ideal weight, your body—being the self-regulating machine that it is—will stop losing weight. I know this sounds unbelievable, but it's true: One woman who did the cleanse for an extraordinary 372 days hit 115 pounds and then stayed at that weight for hundreds of days. (This is not typical.) See the testimonials chapter.

Paradoxically, one friend of mine did the Master Cleanse for 28 days and found that he had *gained* 8 pounds—all of it muscle! The first time I saw him after this cleanse, I could not believe how buffed and chiseled he had become. When he told me that he gained the weight and muscle during his cleanse, I felt awe. This is rare indeed, though I have known extremely thin people to gain as much as a pound in 10 days.

How Long to Stay on the Cleanse

Many people will ask whether they can do a "minicleanse"—say, 3 days of cleansing, or maybe just 5 days. I always stress the importance of doing a minimum of 10 days, for a variety of reasons. Some folks will only do 5 or 6 days of the cleanse and then stop. This is not so good. They have started a process of cleansing that initiates an action to prevent your body from getting sick. If you stop the cleanse too early, the body may take over and make you sick in its attempt to continue the process you originally started, like a boulder rolling down a slope.

The Master Cleanse is a conscious decision to remove toxicity from the body—and getting sick is an unconscious way of attempting to remove toxicity from your body.

In rare cases, I have seen people become sick even after doing 10 days of the cleanse. Such folks need more than the minimum and could likely extend their cleanse by at least another 5 days.

It is interesting to note that many people are so toxic that it might take them 3 or so days for their body to begin the cleansing process. That way they will have at least 7 good days of detox, for a full 10 days of cleansing. This is important, because when you have experienced the many positive changes you get from a minimum of 10 days, you will be motivated to do the cleanse again—and may even make it a part of your lifestyle every few months or so. I occasionally meet people who proudly tell me they have done the Master Cleanse *once*. I ask them, "How was it?" They will say, "It was great." I then ask, "How long ago did you do it?" They say, "Oh, maybe 25 years ago." I respond with "You must be the only person who has ever had sex once!" OK, I

Letting Go of Constipation

Back in the 1980s I was treating a woman in her late 20s who had been suffering from chronic constipation her whole adult life. In our consultation she spoke of her health as a child. She had become so sick from diarrhea that it was life-threatening. It took intense medical intervention to stop the diarrhea and possibly save her. Her health crisis had a deep and long-lasting effect. The constant imprinting to "not let go" or that it might not be safe to let go had come to manifest in her body as constipation. Her unconscious mind was figuratively saving her life by not eliminating. This, of course, led to chronic constipation, which she was treating daily with laxatives.

After I explained to her how the Master Cleanse worked and how to do it, she got on the cleanse ASAP. She did 10 days of the cleanse, and did it properly, seeing me every 3 days or so. She called me right after coming off the cleanse to tell me, worriedly, that she was still constipated. I explained that her condition was not corrected yet and would need more cleansing. She immediately went back on the cleanse for another 10 days and again she called to tell me she was still constipated after 20 days. I reiterated how she still would need more cleansing and eventually her constipation would clear up. She then again know that may be a racy reply, but in fact numerous people have told me that after they complete a Master Cleanse their sex life is just plain better, for they have more energy and aliveness.

How long you stay on the cleanse is entirely up to you. The desired duration is determined by what you have done to yourself in the past, your age, your general health and sense of well-being, and how willing you are to let go of your "stuff." We have many layers of stuff, like an onion, and during a cleanse we peel them away at their own pace. Some layers come off one at a time, and sometimes two or three layers will be stripped away. A few people like to do 40 days at a time, with three or four intervals of rest in between. Some people like to do 10 days at a time every month, for several months. Most people on a regular work or school schedule are happy to be able to do the 10 days in a row.

One big factor for most people is how well they are feeling while on the cleanse. If they feel all right they may want to stay on longer, but if they don't feel so well they may wish to come off. If you are feeling unwell, the middle of a cleanse is a bad time

---

went back on the cleanse, and once more, after about 10 days, she was still constipated. It was becoming apparent that I needed to approach her problem from more than just the physical level. (I was fairly new in my practice and I could have asked about her emotional state much earlier than I was then doing.)

I had expected that the Master Cleanse and the other therapies I was using would successfully address her constipation. But I was now keenly aware that we had to go to the mental and emotional realms and dig up some stuff there. I began by asking her what she was holding onto—maybe she had to let go of something. To my surprise, she started screaming at me in anger, or fear, asking what kind of training I had in psychology, and protesting that I was not qualified to ask such questions. I was unprepared for this onslaught and made an effort to explain myself, but she stopped working with me.

Later, as fate would have it, while shopping in a local health food store I spotted this woman. I felt hesitant about speaking to her, considering our last encounter. I was still expecting her to be angry. Too late! She saw me, came over, and started talking in a friendly manner. We chatted for a few minutes, then I just had to ask "Are you still constipated?" With a big smile she replied, "No!"

to stop. At that point you are at the core of a problem; it is being brought out to show its ugly head so that you can chop it off, so to speak. If you stop too soon, the ugly head will retreat, only to lurk around to pop up later as something like the flu, cold, headache, or any number of other dis-eases.

I have talked to many people who have cleansed for 40 days in a row for religious reasons (echoing the fasts of major spiritual figures). And I have known many people who have done 40 days to overcome various physical challenges that they are experiencing. The longest time I have known to be done in a row is 372 days—just over one solid year; it's an impressive record, in my book! (The second longest was 256 days in a row, or over 36 weeks.)

Women Who Are Pregnant or Nursing

By now you know that the Master Cleanse program supplies enough nutrition to sustain you for at least 10 days without dire consequences. But what about pregnant or nursing women. Don't they have to eat for two? No, not true. I have known even pregnant and nursing mothers to do 10 or more days of the Master Cleanse. My wife nursed two children while doing the cleanse for 7 days, until it became too difficult for her to manage to feed both children, often at the same time. (It still impressed me.)

In 1986 I went to California and spent a week with Stanley Burroughs, my mentor. One night as we watched the local news, a story came on regarding the nutritional requirements for pregnant and nursing women as calculated by a study done at a university in that state. The researchers found that pregnant and nursing women do *not* have to eat for two, because their digestive systems become more efficient and extract more nutrients from their regular diets. Stanley and I just looked at each other and said, "We know that."

If women can do the Master Cleanse safely, then they can also do it safely when they are pregnant or nursing. One friend of mine did the Master Cleanse 5 times in a row for 10 days each, for a total of 50 days, during her pregnancy (with intervals of regular eating in between, of course). Another friend did it 3 times for 10 days each, with no ill effects whatsoever. Both women had quick births and delivered healthy babies.

Children

Can children do the cleanse? How long can they stay on it? I hear this question frequently, because many children today are experiencing dis-ease from the abundance of junk food available and the aggressive marketing campaigns that the advertising industry targets at them. Guidance and support should be sought when dealing with ill or very young children.

One of my fellow classmates in my Vita-Flex class put her 4-month-old granddaughter on the Master Cleanse for 10 days, with no ill effects. I know, I know—send out the authorities. It's curious what many people think is safe for their children. They feed them pounds of sugar and fast food every week, sometimes never even feeding them a fresh vegetable. Their children never exercise, but play video games and watch TV. To me, this is dangerous, but it is deemed the thing to do in our society.

Mom Can Do It Herself

One of my classmates spoke of a friend of hers who put both her 3-year-old and her 5-year-old children on the Master Cleanse for 21 *days!* I later had the pleasure of meeting this woman with her two children shopping in a health food store. I was curious, so I started asking her questions. She explained that her youngest son had been having brain seizures and convulsions and she had exhausted the medical system trying to find answers. There seemed to be none. Doctors simply could not find the problem, and therefore had no solution. She decided to take matters into her own hands and put the two boys onto the Master Cleanse; she would do it too, along with them. On Day 10 the youth authorities showed up at her door, because someone had reported her for starving her boys. She invited them in to observe her boys' health and behavior, while she explained her dilemma and her reasons for using the Master Cleanse. The authorities eventually left, satisfied that the children were both healthy and happy. I then asked how her youngest son was now, and she said that he had not had any seizures since doing the Master Cleanse. It may have been only three or four months since they all finished the cleanse.

The Elderly

The oldest person whom I have witnessed doing the Master Cleanse was 94 years of age. She did quite well and had few, if any, problems while doing it. Nevertheless, I stress the importance of monitoring elderly people while cleansing, and making sure that they follow all the necessary steps to ensure success.

Keep an Eye on Your Tongue   I decided during my Stanley Burroughs training that I would cleanse until my tongue got pink. I had learned that the tongue is a barometer to the body's toxicity, just as a weather vane tells you which way the wind is blowing. When you start cleansing, the tongue will turn white and become coated. After several days it will start to turn pink at the edges and the plaque on it will recede from the front to the back of the tongue. (You cannot simply brush your tongue pink after 6 days and then say you are done!) The progress of my own tongue after 16 days made me decide to cleanse in short lengths of 10 to 15 days at a time. It took me about 100 days in the year to feel as good off the cleanse as I did while on it.

How to End the Master Cleanse

Whether you are old or young, or in between, to complete the Master Cleanse you must come off the lemonade diet properly. *I cannot overemphasize this point.* I have known many people to eat food too soon after a cleanse, or too much food, or the wrong kind. For some people, of course, their biggest pleasure in life is food. Ask yourself whether you live to eat or eat to live, and pay attention to your answer.

The important transition period of moving from lemonade to food will prepare your digestive system for more and more complex foods so that it does not become overwhelmed. Just as you wouldn't try running a marathon after being a couch potato for three years, you wouldn't break a cleanse by launching into full-feasting mode. You want your digestive system to get a well-deserved break so that your body can start back on the right track.

You have done 10 or more days of cleansing. Please continue to treat your body with the respect it deserves. Why not give yourself a pat on the back for completing 10 full days of lemonade. Now you can come off the lemonade diet in one of two ways: eating a vegetarian diet, or eating a normal diet.

Vegetarian (or Vegan) Diet

Let's say that you are already a vegetarian, or perhaps even a complete vegan. To my mind, this is the best of all possible worlds for your health.

Days 1 and 2 after you complete your Master Cleanse
Drink only freshly squeezed orange juice throughout the day. You can eat whole oranges during this period as well. Drink the juice slowly, taking time to relish the taste. Some people might want to dilute the orange juice with water for one day, to make the transition easier.

I have dealt with probably fewer than 20 people who could not stand having orange juice after the lemonade. This is not dependent on whether or not they could drink orange juice before the Master Cleanse, just something peculiar to their system. In those cases I suggested that they eat fresh papaya, and add fresh pineapple and fresh mango for variety. These same foods make the adjustment to a regular diet easier. In extreme cases, people coming off the cleanse could tolerate no fruit at all, and could only consume vegetable soup broth for a few days.

Day 3   Have fresh orange juice in the morning and eat fruit salad for lunch. I make a dressing with a bit of orange juice, pineapple chunks, and papaya slices in the blender, to top the fruit salad. Enjoy fruit or (uncooked) vegetable salad in the evening.

Day 4   You can now start your normal eating of a vegetarian or vegan diet.

Regular ("Normal") Diet

The second way to come off a cleanse is designed for those people who have not followed an optimal diet throughout their life.

(Eating junk foods, processed foods, and animal food products fits this so-called normal category.)

Day 1 Drink fresh-squeezed orange juice all day. Drink several glasses of it, diluted with water if necessary.

Day 2 Drink fresh orange juice again throughout the day. Prepare a vegetable soup in the afternoon, or when possible, and consume only the broth, with just a small amount of vegetables in it. Enjoy the soup for dinner. The soup is to be made from as many fresh vegetables as you can find. In the winter, when fresh vegetables are not plentiful, I like to include a few frozen items, such as peas and corn. Do not use meat or meat stock; use dehydrated vegetable powders instead. Add spices and sea salt to taste. Do not overcook the vegetables until they are limp; you want as much good nourishment as possible.

Day 3 Continue to drink fresh orange juice in the morning, and also have some during the day if you wish. Have vegetable soup for lunch, this time eating all the vegetables you have added to the soup. In the evening, eat a vegetable salad with a light dressing. For the main course, eat brown rice or quinoa with steamed vegetables, which will taste like heaven. Learn to appreciate simple meals with fewer animal proteins. Start reading cookbooks with a wider variety of vegetable dishes. Expand your repertoire of foods and your palate, but wisely.

You have finished the Master Cleanse. Good for you! Always acknowledge your successes, and take the best from all the rest.

Special Situations

Everyone wants to be special—but trust me, you are not! I have had people do a successful Master Cleanse even though they had parts of their colon removed, or had had their bladder removed, or were missing their spleen, or were deaf, or blind, or given a week to live, or needed bypass surgery, or had no gall bladder or appendix, or had birth defects, or serious iatrogenic conditions, mental disorders, addictions...and on and on. The variety of conditions I have helped treat is truly staggering, and the successes reported back to me are even more so. If you really think you have a special situation, please just reread this book, then do the cleanse.

The most common problem I hear from people is that they are *hypoglycemic;* that is, they suffer from low blood sugar or energy crashes. This condition comes from eating too much sugar or processed foods, or (as some people believe) from feeling a lack of sweetness in life or having a "What's the use?!" attitude. I rarely see anyone these days who does not have a few hypoglycemic symptoms. People in this condition must keep their energy up by drinking several glasses of the special lemonade drink each day—maybe as much as 12 or more in total for the first 3 days or so—before cutting back.

Candida problems are another reason that people think they cannot do the Master Cleanse. (Refer to Chapter 5 for more information.) Apparently, sugar causes *Candida* to grow in your body. The only fuel your body burns is sugar; you must have sugar in your bloodstream or you will die. The problem with *Candida* is that it creates overacidity. A compromised colon wall will then leak *Candida* into the blood. We have to reduce the irritation of the lining of the colon and alkalize the body, at the same time. This does not always work fast enough on the cleanse to contain *Candida* growth, so some people (though not all) will experience an increase of their symptoms. To counteract this problem, they can take GSE (grapefruit seed extract) or oregano essential oil in capsules. (See Chapter 9 for details.) You will have to determine the number of drops per capsule for your own needs. If you take the extra steps to deal with the *Candida,* you can benefit from the Master Cleanse.

People suffering from *fibromyalgia* will almost always feel worse the entire 10 days, and maybe into a second cleanse as well. They will feel better when they stop the cleanse, but it's vital that they do several cleanses in a row in order to affect the fibromyalgia. Taking a product with the highest quality MSM (methylsulfonylmethane, a bioavailable and hypoallergenic form of sulfur) for two weeks before the cleanse can prevent this. If that does not work, the cause is the poor quality of the MSM.

Stanley Burroughs recommended that people on *medications* wean themselves off them over 3 to 4 days, then possibly go back on their medication, though at a reduced dosage. You will want to check this out with your doctor, in advance, to determine how best to deal with your medications after a cleanse.

Stanley gives special instructions for *insulin-dependent diabetics* in his book *Healing for the Age of Enlightenment*.

People with *transplants* or those taking *immune-suppressant drugs* cannot do the Master Cleanse, as detailed earlier in this chapter.

Repeat this mantra: "When in doubt, follow the instructions."

What to Expect After the Master Cleanse

Now that you have completed the cleanse, what do you do next? Sit back and just enjoy how you're feeling now? Compare your results with the list of benefits that began this chapter, just for fun and to feel a sense of satisfaction? These are questions that people ask themselves, and for good reason.

Some folks may want to go back to the life they led before the Master Cleanse. This reminds me about a medical study that found that when the heart beat became very regular and predictable, then a heart attack was soon to occur. Similarly, when the brain was monitored and its waves became highly regular and predictable, that's the time that petit mal seizures would occur. This was an enlightening study for some, but not necessarily for others who are more aware of how the universe works. In my way of thinking, the universe, the world, and our own personal lives all exist in an ever-changing environment. If we are not changing or failing to adapt to the new circumstance in our lives, we are in fact dying, by degrees. It appears that change is not only good for us but a *must* for us to stay healthy. Yet change for change's sake is not always the best thing.

After each of my own cleanses, I have found that my body felt much more attuned and sensitive to what I ate. I was no longer numb to its urging, as I had been before, and mindlessly eating whatever was put in front of me. In the past, when I got very busy I would ignore my body's signal to eliminate, and would find myself becoming constipated. In response to this tendency, I now immediately go to the bathroom whenever I feel the urge to have a bowel movement. I also became a vegetarian after the first time I did the Master Cleanse because it simply felt better to eat differently and more healthfully. (A few years ago I consumed seafood now and then.)

I am sometimes amused by those people who initially tell me that they do not want to change their lifestyle, then do a Master Cleanse and quickly change their mind and tell me about it excitedly. They find that their old lifestyle no longer has the same appeal or worthiness. Truly, it is hard to go back to a lifestyle that may not ultimately be good for your health. The Master Cleanse can make this painfully obvious.

How to Eat After the Cleanse

I used to give my clients a list of rules about how they "should" eat after they come off the Master Cleanse. This was extremely dogmatic of me, and not always the most effective way to encourage people I cared about to make positive changes. These days, I suggest to my clients that they start changing slowly—by introducing certain foods into their daily diets, and leaving other ones alone. They can then make their own assessments from what they eat and how they feel and how they look afterward. This program turns out to be a far more empowering experience, and produces better results than turning their eating practices around 180 degrees.

I typically offer a number of basic suggestions:

Eat raw foods, as much as possible. They are high in enzymes, which makes them easier to digest, assimilate, and then eliminate. (See the chart of alkaline and acidic foods on the facing page.)

Eat an alkaline diet, one that is at least 80 percent alkaline forming to the body.

Avoid processed foods as much as you possibly can—those containing white flour, white sugar, white rice, white vinegar, and the like.

Go organic whenever possible. (Many supermarket chains are expanding their product line of organic offerings.) Organic foods almost always taste better than nonorganic, and besides that they contain more nutrients and are more ecofriendly. Eat locally when you can!

Drink plenty of pure water throughout the day. This will help you absorb nutrients more effectively and will assist your cells in their task of dumping toxins and flushing out your system on a daily basis.

Beware the nightshade. Many people feel better when they avoid plants in the nightshade family of herbs, shrubs, and trees. Cayenne, of course, is an exception to this rule and is used in the lemonade. Tomatoes, potatoes, eggplant, peppers, and tobacco belong in this group. (Belladonna, or medical atropine, is extracted from the "deadly nightshade" plant.)

To expand on the last item above: Foods from the nightshade family tend to exacerbate any inflammatory conditions you might have. They may also cause headaches and trigger migraines in some people. I have had clients grow angry when I tell them that they may have been sickened by eating these popular foods. I first ask them whether they love to eat these foods, and they reply "Yes." I then ask whether they have specific symptoms, and again they reply in the affirmative. At that point I tell them, "So, connect the dots. You eat these foods and you have these problems, so figure it out—cause and effect." I remind them of one more

ALKALINE AND ACID-FORMING FOODS

When attempting to alkalize your body, it is important to remember that it is the effect in the body of a particular food you must consider. For example, though lemons are highly acid, their effect on the body when they are consumed is to alkalize it. Generally, all fruits, vegetables, and sprouts as well as their juice, when fresh or raw, are alkalizing to the body.

You should avoid or minimize foods that form acid in the body when you are cleansing. Almost all processed foods are acid-forming in the body.

The lists below are not complete but give examples of regularly consumed foods in each of the categories. Many good books and websites are available to further your knowledge in this area.

Foods That Alkalize the Body

Apples
Apricots
Bananas (yellow)
Beets & their greens
Berries
Blackberries
Broccoli
Cabbage
Cantaloupe
Carrots
Cauliflower
Celery
Cherries
Coconut
Dates
Grapefruits
Grapes
Green beans
Kale
Kelp
Leaf lettuce
Lemons
Limes
Mangoes
Olive oil (organic cold-pressed)
Onions
Oranges
Parsley
Peaches
Pears
Pineapple
Radishes
Raisins
Raspberries
Sauerkraut
Spinach
Squash
Yams
Watermelon

Foods That Form Acid in the Body

Alcohol
Baked bread
Cake
Canned or processed fruits & vegetables
Cereals (all)
Chocolate
Coffee
Cooked grains
Dairy
Eggs
Foods cooked with oils
Fruits that have been glazed or sulfured
Ketchup
Legumes
Lentils & beans (dried)
Nuts (most)
Meat, poultry, shellfish
Pasta
Pepper (black)
Popcorn
Salt
Soft drinks
Soy products
Sugar (white & processed)
Sweeteners, artificial
Tea (black)
Vinegar, distilled
Wheat (all forms)

factor related to their experience of these foods: that is, how much water they drink every day while eating foods from the nightshade family. I remind them that the more water they drink, the less noticeable their discomfort will be. I give them a simple test: Eat nothing from the nightshade family for at least two weeks; then eat from among these foods at all three meals for one day only, while paying close attention to how their body feels for the next 24 hours or so. They will have their answer, tailored to their own body's chemistry.

If you take in all the above suggestions of what to do after your cleanse, you are not exactly doing rocket science. Instead, you are using common sense and learning to become more aware of your body. You are perhaps dredging up memories of what you have done to it over the years, and you are starting to put the puzzle pieces together. Routinely in my practice, I find that many clients come to me with maybe the borders of their life-puzzle filled in. I simply help them put the remaining pieces in place, so that they can see the big picture of their health choices. Doing this with them, rather than for them, makes it much easier to help them understand what is happening in their life, and how to make the choices that work best *for them*.

Improving Your Health in Other Ways

- Do weight or strength training, and combine it with cardiovascular training.
- Do yoga, Pilates, tai chi, gentle martial arts, BOSU®, or other nonextreme body work.
- Practice relaxation.
- Learn meditation.
- Practice mindful living.
- Love yourself unconditionally.
- Use a shower filter to remove chlorine.
- Choose a job you enjoy, or change the job you have to make it more satisfying.

- Find activities that help you experience fulfillment or joy.
- Become a foster parent, adopt a child, or mentor a troubled youth.
- Offer one hour a week to an elderly neighbor who will enjoy your company and might have you do small projects.
- Stop using shampoo and soaps containing sodium lauryl sulfate and similar compounds.
- Cease using skin care products with preservatives or synthetic compounds, including perfumes.
- Do not use a microwave oven.
- Practice forgiveness.
- Start a gratitude journal.
- Choose friends who love and support you...and love them back.

Enhancing Your Results

I have amassed a number of suggestions of things to help you optimize your results from the Master Cleanse and lock in mechanisms for success.

1. Read this entire book before starting your cleanse. Many people take the shortcut of reading only the basic instruction portion of the book. This means that they have not absorbed all the information offered, and therefore are ill prepared when questions or difficulties arise.

2. Pick 10 days to do the cleanse, marking them on your calendar or day-planner. Choose dates when you have little or no social engagements, and minimal travel requirements. It is too cruel to attend a dinner function and not be eating. It is even harder on the cleanse to go to the home of friends if your activities will be centered on eating or drinking alcohol. Plan activities that do not involve eating. Go on a hike, find a different community pool and go swimming, or rent a rowboat and spend a peaceful hour or two in the park. Renting movies on DVD will be easier than attending cineplexes, where people will be munching and gulping all around you. Cut back on watching TV, which can be difficult because of all the enticing food commercials.

3. Negotiate with your spouse or partner for them to do the cooking and grocery shopping for themselves and your children during the entire 10 days of your cleanse. Focus on yourself for a change.

4. Plan to start the cleanse on the weekend or when you have several consecutive days off work. Most people find the first few days the hardest. Choose not to do the cleanse over a holiday. It is pretty hard not to eat food while everyone else is enjoying a lovely Thanksgiving feast.

5. Line up your supporters. Think about those among your friends and family who will be most supportive of you, then arrange to spend time with them. Stay away from people who will sabotage you. Tell only those people who will support you that you are doing a cleanse. Don't listen to negative expressions.

6. Gather your ingredients in advance. If possible, buy only organic lemons, limes, and oranges. Ripen your fruit by letting it sit out on the counter for a few days before you use it. Buy your sea salt and herbal laxative. The salt must be sea salt, not regular salt, and not the iodized kind. All these items can be found at health food stores or in the natural section of many grocery stores or supermarkets.

7. If you drink coffee or caffeinated sodas, or eat chocolate or sugary foods on a daily basis, try to wean yourself away from these foods before starting the cleanse.

8. Remember that you can use herbal remedies such as ginger for stomach upset or drinking peppermint tea if your breath is bad. If you have an herbalist available, consult them about using herbal remedies while cleansing, but don't let them discourage you from doing the cleanse. Remember that you can drink herbal teas that don't contain caffeine, for both pleasure and variety.

9. Start a cleansing journal, like the one on pages 190–91. Write in it your goals, why you are doing the cleanse, what you hope to achieve from it, and who your support partner is. Keep track of what you do and how you feel. Each day, keep track of how much lemonade you drink, whether you eliminate or not,

and how you feel emotionally. If you run into a problem, it will be easier to figure out what the issue is when you can consult your journal. At the end of your cleanse, write down your results and any things you want to try on your next cleanse.

10. Prepare yourself both mentally and emotionally. Set a date to start the cleanse, and then consider what issues might come up for you. Look for solutions to those problems, and gather support to help you overcome them. Support could be in the form of information or the ability to use some adjunct therapy. It also could be in the form of someone else who has done the Master Cleanse, or a practitioner of Vita-Flex, or someone else well versed in the work of Stanley Burroughs or other holistic healers. It could be a massage therapist or Reflexologist who will support you in doing the cleanse. If you anticipate significant problems, find a practitioner early on who can help you if and when necessary, including a phone consultation if needed. Not all alternative therapists support cleansing, mostly because they have not done it themselves and are unaware of the benefits of doing the Master Cleanse.

11. Make sure that if you feel tired you get lots of rest.

12. Find something inspiring to read during your cleanse. There are lots of motivating and helpful books to read that can support you in changing and healing your life. While cleansing, avoid magazines that feature tempting food ads, recipes, and other "eye candy."

13. Use affirmations to promote your healing. Write your favorite ones down, and post them on your bathroom mirror. Read them aloud several times a day. Here are a few examples:

—I am willing to change.

—I find success in all my endeavors

—It is safe for me to cleanse.

—I release the need to be ill.

—I always feel supported on my path to wellness.

—I am becoming healthier and happier day by day.

14. Wear bright-colored clothes. Spend time in the sunshine and breath in the fresh air, and out with the old.

15. Listen to inspiring music or watch edifying movies that depict positive changes, not violence or special effects.

16. Use the time that you are not spending to shop for, prepare, and cook your normal foods as an opportunity to clean up your external life. While you are doing the Master Cleanse you can tackle easy chores like primping or cleaning up your body (nails, hair, skin, calluses), tidying up your bedroom or workroom, sorting your papers, and getting small tasks out of the way.

17. Consider following an exercise program. Start lightly, at first. You could begin by just walking 30 minutes a day, then working up to a longer or more vigorous walk.

18. Do yoga.

19. Meditate.

20. Use an herbal remedy during the Master Cleanse to help rid yourself of internal parasites. (See Chapter 11 for details.)

21. Take a sauna and or use a steam room to assist the detoxification process. Infrared saunas, if available in your area, are the least stressful to the heart and the most efficient type of sauna to maximize the healing process.

Avoiding Common Mistakes

At the risk of being repetitive, I have gathered the most typical mistakes that people make on a cleanse. You might use this as a checklist for what *NOT* to do:

- Not preparing mentally for the cleanse or not reading the instructions first.
- Not drinking adequate amounts of lemonade each day.
- Waiting until too late in the day before drinking the first glass of lemonade. Drink it within the first several hours after you wake up.
- Drinking more water than lemonade during the cleanse.

- Not drinking the lemonade fresh. Or not making the drink up in large quantities or in advance. *Note:* Only use a concentrate when you absolutely have to.
- Taking the ingredients separately. Or omitting one ingredient altogether. *Tip:* The body needs the combination of ingredients to maximize cleansing.
- Not drinking the lemonade within 10 minutes of preparation.
- Not taking the herbal laxative every night and every morning, if you choose not to do the salt water flush. *Solution:* Adjust the amount of laxative you take by steeping the laxative tea longer or taking more capsules if you are not eliminating enough. Decrease the laxative if you are overly cramping or are eliminating way too much. Increase the amount of salt if the salt water does not pass out through the rectum when doing the internal salt water flush.
- Worrying about being on the cleanse needlessly. *Good news:* In 10 days you will neither starve nor fade away like the Cheshire cat!
- Not using ripe lemon or limes.
- Not using the best possible pure water.
- Using honey or any other sweetener, except as outlined in this book or in Stanley Burroughs's books.
- Cheating. *Tip:* Eating even small amounts of anything other than the approved ingredients will affect the success of your Master Cleanse. Do not accept so much as a forkful of dessert from your companion.
- Stopping too soon.
- Using 2 tablespoons of salt, rather than 2 *teaspoons*, when mixing the salt water bath.
- Continuing with supplements while on the cleanse.
- Putting cayenne in the concentrate. *Caution:* Doing so will make it "steep" and result in lemonade that is way too hot. Instead, add the cayenne to the drink as you prepare it.
- Coming off the cleanse improperly.

PART 3

Adjuncts to the Master Cleanse

CHAPTER 7

Vita-Flex,
to Balance the Body

To support the results of a Master Cleanse, Stanley Burroughs practiced a second modality, which he called Vita-Flex. This is a technique of physical manipulation that can support and make more effective the use of the cleanse and give vitality to the system. I have been able to help many thousands of people while on a cleanse by giving them Vita-Flex treatments. Treatments can relieve pain, help balance hormones, relax the body, and do so much more. Results can be accomplished often in mere seconds, or minutes at the most.

Vita-Flex is a reflexive, or pressure point, massage technique that Stanley rediscovered in the late 1920s through an intuitive insight. He told me that one day he suddenly saw himself, in his mind's eye, employing this reflex massage on someone. He could even see the charts of the various reflex points for the entire body. The technique is believed to have been developed in Tibet over 5,000 years ago, and even predates acupuncture. Tibetan lamas even told Stanley personally that people in Tibet practice this technique (and possibly still do today).

Vita-Flex is similar to Reflexology, though is a more extensive and comprehensive therapy because it is applied throughout many more areas of the body. The Vita-Flex technique is slightly different and more effective than Reflexology. Many Reflexologists whom I have taught would agree with me. Stanley coined the name Vita-Flex because it denoted health or vitality gained through the reflexes. The word *reflex* is derived from *reflexive,* meaning "to direct back onto one's self." A person who does Vita-Flex is activating the inborn system of bodily reflexes to correct or balance the body by its own natural means.

In this and the following several chapters, I will share a number of stories from my own practice and from Stanley's as well.

The Basics of Vita-Flex

Vita-Flex is a technique in which the thumb, middle, and index fingers are used one at a time to stimulate or activate various pressure points on the body. The fingers or thumb rotate 180 degrees over the contacted skin by the fingertip. This manipulation looks similar to a blended movement of, say, pulling the trigger of a gun and rotating your hand as if you are turning a door knob.

This manipulation causes what is called a piezoelectric effect, or electric polarity caused by pressure (sometimes in a crystalline substance, such as quartz). This effect happens when a mechanical movement by the therapist induces an electrical release of energy by the recipient. This energy does *not* come from the person applying Vita-Flex but instead is generated by the person receiving the treatment.

Pick Yourself Up

One day, while visiting Stanley, I was present as a young woman who came to his house limped over to him in severe pain after falling off a horse. Her mount had thrown her onto rocks and she had landed on them, hard, with heavy camera gear in her backpack. I watched as Stanley did about 20 minutes of Vita-Flex on this woman. By the end she was twisting and turning her body to try and find the very last iota of discomfort so that Stanley could alleviate it with his fingers. It was truly a blessing for me to watch him perform—and, of course, a blessing for her to receive such a beneficial treatment.

This electrical energy does not travel along nerves in the body, but travels on an entirely different system altogether. In some systems of healing, these pathways are referred to as meridians. Stanley said these Vita-Flex pathways have not been identified yet because they were so minuscule and they dissolve in the body quickly after death.

The Body's Reflex Points

In this system of therapy, the body is understood to have well over 1,500 reflex points on it. Many of them are concentrated in five main areas: feet, hands, ears, scalp, and face. It is on these areas that the whole map of the body is displayed, and during a Vita-Flex treatment all five are activated. The ears, being so small, are an exception; they are instead rubbed between the fingers to stimulate circulation in the body. Interestingly, this physical fact may have been the reason that acupuncture was developed: A fingertip is too large to effectively access the reflex points in the ears, so someone had the idea to use instead a pointed instrument—hence the acupuncture needle, which has an honorable cultural history.

One unique aspect of Vita-Flex is that a single reflex point can affect more than one area of the body. In fact, because we are three-dimensional beings, Vita-Flex will work through all three dimensions. For example, it will work from the feet up into the body, and it will also work from the front of the body to the back and vice versa. Lastly, it will work from one side of the body to the other.

The advantage to this is that many reflex points are available to address one specific point in the body. Another advantage to a reflexive massage is that it enables the practitioner to work directly (but reflexively) on an injured or diseased area without causing pain or further injury. Using this therapy a practitioner can affect organs, glands, and even whole systems in the body with an application of this noninvasive technique.

The Vita-Flex technique uses the body's own self-regulating or balancing process and supports the body in its own healing.

The techniques will never overstimulate, because the reflex points on the body can be stimulated only five or six times before they stop responding. They are like a cup being filled with water; once the cup is full, it will hold no more water, no matter how much is poured into it. The unique aspects of this technique make this therapy simple, extremely effective, and easily applied.

As the situation required, I have done treatments in airport lounges, homes, hospitals, restaurants, nursing homes, and rehabilitation facilities, to cite only a few locations where I have done Vita-Flex.

Over the years I have found the technique to be useful and effective on many types and conditions of people, from newborn babies to people well into their 90s, and from healthy persons to extremely ill ones.

Treatment Technique Described

The technique is quite simple, but it does take practice to perfect. It is described by Stanley as pulling the trigger of a gun while rotating your wrist at the same time. Generally, only the index finger, middle finger, or the thumb is used to apply Vita-Flex. One digit is used at a time. The practitioner also has to anchor the thumb or fingers on the body while applying the technique, so he or she uses an appropriate pressure as the fingertip rolls or moves over the reflex point. In fact, the last joint of the finger will rotate 180 degrees if the technique is properly done.

While the written description of this technique appears complicated, the technique is really quite simple to understand when visually observed. In other words, best seen to be understood.

Vita-Flex was created long before massage tables were designed. Therefore, a Vita-Flex session has long been done, successfully, with both the practitioner and the recipient in a seated position. The recipient removes shoes and usually socks. No equipment or supplies whatsoever are required. Peace, warmth, and quiet create a good atmosphere for treatment. Some contemporary massage therapists will incorporate Vita-Flex during a massage on a table, though using a table does not work well for a complete session. A full Vita-Flex treatment takes 40 minutes to one hour, depending on the recipient's condition and concerns.

The Atlas Adjustment

Most applications of Vita-Flex are free of pain. One exception may be noted: an application called the Atlas Adjustment. It is aptly named. You may recall that in Greek mythology Atlas, a Titan who joined in a revolt against the gods, was forced by Zeus to bear the heavens on his shoulders. We too support the most important things in our personal world—our brain, mind, and soul—on top of our spine.

This application is utilized to correct a misalignment of the top vertebra. Stanley believed that the structural alignment of a person's body is determined early in life by the placement of the Atlas, or first cervical vertebra. If a person's Atlas is misaligned, the commands for the placement of all the other vertebrae below are compromised. The spine often then distorts, to some degree, which forces the body to compensate by tilting the pelvis. People with this misalignment may suffer headaches or have neck, back, hip, or knee pain—to name only a few symptoms.

The Atlas Adjustment is done with no manipulation or adjustment of the spine, but is completed by firmly pressing two reflex points on the clavicle near the AC joint (where the shoulder blade meets the collarbone). Some people may experience an intense but temporary pain where the thumb applies a quick, deep pressure; it lasts for only seconds.

My own first experience with Vita-Flex occurred in front of an audience on January 7, 1980. My teacher, Maynard Dalderis, was doing an introductory talk on Vita-Flex, Color Therapy, and the Master Cleanse. As he started to describe the Atlas Adjustment to the audience, I couldn't resist, so I shot my arm up and implored him, "Do me, do me!" Maynard said I could come up at the end of the talk and he would demonstrate this technique on me.

At that time of my life I was experiencing severe headaches, accompanied by intense neck and shoulder pain. I had suffered at least three severe injuries in my neck and shoulder, from playing football, and I had been seeing a specialist. My doctor showed me X-rays of my neck where vertebrae C3 and C4, along with C6 and C7, showed a severe buildup of calcium. The doctor prescribed painkillers, which I refused to take unless the pain lasted for more than three days at a time. The only other option he offered me was to have these two cervical vertebrae areas fused together to stop the pain, which would mean that I would lose a great deal of mobility in my neck. Talk about being between a rock and a hard place! What a choice I had.

At the end of his talk, Maynard invited me to the front of the audience to demonstrate the Atlas Adjustment on me.

Visualize this as best you can: The person receiving the technique is sat down properly by the practitioner, who guides them squarely onto a chair; they cannot be twisted at all to either side. The person's legs are then lifted and measured on the inside part of the legs at the ankle bone to see whether one leg is longer than the other. If one leg is found to be shorter, then it is on that side that the reflex point is first pressed along the collarbone. Then the other side is done immediately afterward.

I can vividly recall the details of my own first treatment, those many years ago when I was trying to find my calling and was learning about a variety of health issues and physical treatments. My teacher, Maynard, sat me down properly in a chair and measured my legs. It turned out that my left leg was about ¾ inch shorter than my right. In fact, my left leg was not actually shorter; my left hip was *higher* than my right one.

I already knew that there was something unusual with my body because I tended to wear down the tread on the bottom of my left shoe completely but still have about half the tread remaining on

Wrestler's Neck and an Atlas Adjustment

One weekend I was away with my daughter at a wrestling competition. This sport is intense, and it is not uncommon for several injuries to occur over the course of a weekend meet. I had left the auditorium for a time and when I returned several people were kneeling around someone lying on one of the mats. After what seemed to be 30 minutes they finally moved the injured athlete and I recognized him as a young man who shared the same coach as my daughter. So I immediately went to that coach and offered my assistance. He took me to the area where the young man had been taken, away from the crowd. I told the wrestler that I could perhaps help him, if he wished it. He indicated that he would like my help and that it was OK for me to try my best. It turned out that he had been picked up and dropped onto his head and injured his neck. He was sitting up but not able to turn his neck without much pain.

my right shoe. People also would tell me that I was easily identifiable by my odd gait, even when they saw me from a distance.

Maynard applied pressure, first on my left side and then on my right side. I was told to stand up and walk about, then I came back to the chair and was sat down once again to be remeasured. This second measuring showed that I had adjusted my short-leg length disparity by about 50 percent. Great news! But it meant that the technique had to be reapplied. When Maynard applied the pressure a second time, I felt what seemed to be an intense electrical shock go from my left shoulder to my left hip, and my shorter left leg lurched forward suddenly.

I stood up and walked, came back to the chair, and was sat down properly. Then I was remeasured, and this time we found that either both legs were the same length or my hips were realigned—it made no difference which happened (it was six of one, half a dozen of the other, in effect). It has been 27 years since that memorable treatment, almost to the day, as I write this. And my neck and shoulders are still well. True, I occasionally get a stiff neck, probably from sleeping crookedly or napping without proper neck support, but usually a few minutes of Vita-Flex that I do on myself will alleviate it.

I told him I would do Vita-Flex for his neck by doing an Atlas Adjustment. I also warned him that it might be uncomfortable for him when I pushed on the two points near his collarbone to accomplish this. I pressed one point quite deeply and he seemed to cry silently for several seconds, and then I repeated the process on the other side. He cried again and after a few seconds I told him to try to move his head. He was still afraid to turn his neck, but the more he turned it the more surprised he looked. He now had his head turned completely to one side and he said that all the pain in his neck was gone. I asked him if he had any other pain, and he said that he had a headache (quite normal, considering his being dropped on his head). I quickly did the headache points too, and he then said his headache was also gone.

All this occurred in less than two minutes. He then got up normally and left the room. Later he was seen running and wrestling with his friends. Case closed!

After my first experience with Vita-Flex, I thought it was a very simple but effective technique that could activate my body's own balancing or regulating mechanisms. To my wonderment, that first adjustment lasted until late August 1988, or more than eight years, at which time I got into a bicycle accident and suffered several injuries. I was not wearing a helmet in those days, and I struck my head on the pavement and cut my head open. Such a shock is more than enough to put the Atlas out of alignment. But I had to continue working.

Two days later, when I was about to do an Atlas Adjustment on a client (who happened to be a massage therapist), I quipped that my Atlas had *really* shrugged and that I myself badly needed an adjustment on it. He asked me to demonstrate how to do it on him, and then he did an Atlas Adjustment on me, successfully, to my great relief.

Correcting a Prolapsed Colon

The prolapsed colon lift is another technique developed by Stanley Burroughs. It consists of simply moving a prolapsed (or fallen) colon back to its proper resting position in the abdominal cavity.

The colon falls down usually as a result of poor diet, lack of exercise (which creates poor muscle tone of the abdominal muscles), and a failure to cleanse the colon regularly. In my many years of experience I have seen fewer than 10 people who did *not* have some degree of a prolapsed colon. Unfortunately, most people have severe problems with their colon, which has many impacts on their health.

A colon that is twisted or folded, kinked or congested, will not effectively dump waste matter or be cleansed properly while on the lemonade diet—or on any other diet, for that matter. When a woman's colon falls, it will lie on her uterus, ovaries, and bladder, causing a host of conditions and problems. (See illustrations below.) I believe that many reproductive problems can be reversed with extensive cleansing and moving the colon up to its normal position—then keeping it there.

For both women *and* men, this is an important aspect of properly cleansing the body. If your own colon is not in its nat-

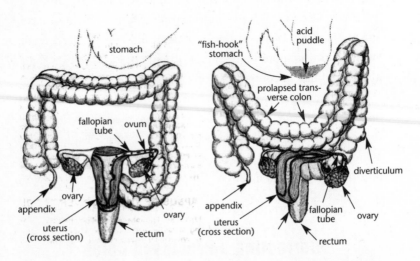

*Left: Normal colon and uterus. Note normal position of stomach. **Right:** Prolapsed colon with pressure on uterus. Note that ovum cannot transit fallopian tube due to pressure. Uterus cannot pass menstrual discharge efficiently. Prolapsus of transverse colon allows stomach to drop—resulting in "fish-hook" stomach.*

ural position, it cannot cleanse itself completely. If such cleansing is prevented, your body will not detoxify at the cellular level as effectively as possible. Unfortunately for everybody, at present very few people in North America know how to correct a prolapsed colon. I am hopeful, however, that health practitioners and holistic healers will be motivated to learn the technique.

Finding Treatment and Relief

At this point, you might be wondering where you can find someone to do these therapies on you. Sad to say, few qualified Vita-Flex practitioners are readily available. Luckily, there is one option for people who cannot find a practitioner. Stanley invented a massage tool that would effectively imitate Vita-Flex on the feet and body.

I asked him many years ago whether he would allow me to manufacture this product, because I believed it was the best reflex massage aide of its type. He said yes. This product is called the Relax-a-Roller. It is available mostly online, but in addition is sold by some Reflexologists, massage therapists, and chiropractors. It is also available through some retail outlets.

Educational Resources

To assist students, not only do I teach workshops on the Vita-Flex technique, but also I have created a DVD on which I demonstrate how to do Vita-Flex with the most accurate technique possible, given the absence of personal hands-on training.

To learn more about Vita-Flex, read Stanley Burroughs's book *Healing for the Age of Enlightenment* or view my DVD (titled "Vita-Flex: The Instructional Video with Tom Woloshyn"), or do both.

You can also visit my website—www.vitagem.com—for information about my teaching schedule, to purchase the DVD, to find a practitioner in your area, or to learn about other products and resources available.

CHAPTER 8

Color Therapy,
to Optimize Light's Energy

The first therapy that Stanley Burroughs practiced was Color Therapy. He was taught it in 1925 or 1926 by Dinshah Ghadiali (who later became known as Colonel Dinshah). Color Therapy is simply the shining or application of specific frequencies or colors of light onto the body to bring about its healing or balance. For example, if you have a "hot condition," such as a fever, burn, or infection, you would shine a cool color on the body to create balance.

On several occasions over the last 25 years I have gotten sunburned. This is a hot condition and to treat it successfully you apply the color turquoise onto your body for at least 1 hour, then wait at least 2 hours before applying another color. When I have done this the burn and pain has disappeared with just one or two applications of Color Therapy. Even when the burn was on my back I would shine light on the front of my body and it would still work.

You may be skeptical of what I have just described; I myself felt that way when I first read about it.

The Ancient Roots of Color Therapy

As I learned from Stanley, the principles of Color Therapy were written in hieroglyphics on the great pyramids of Egypt. The ancient Romans and Greeks also used the practice. I was taught that, long before stained glass windows were made as works of religious art, the use of Color Therapy was commonly practiced in churches. Some churches even held small booths or enclosures constructed of stained glass panes that people would go into and pray for healing. Indeed, the stained glass windows we now enjoy viewing in churches and cathedrals were originally inspired by the practice of Color Therapy.

In 2006, I was in Spain touring a number of churches with an architect friend. As we walked through one church, she noted that in her historical research she had found that Color Therapy was done in churches before the rise of stained glass windows. A study had even been done on the apparent spontaneous healings of people while attending church. It found that the individuals who had experienced this phenomenon had one thing in common—they were all sitting in the light pouring through the stained glass windows.

But how can shining light on your body affect your health, or anything else, for that matter? Think about it from a larger perspective. If there were no light on Planet Earth, would there be any life here? Most likely not. In fact, we are light beings, and electrical beings. You might be surprised to learn that our bodies generate about as much light as a 75-watt bulb. We cannot see this light, however, because it is in the infrared range of invisible radiation wavelengths. Yet we can sense the light as heat.

Police, firefighters, military troops, and rescue teams all use infrared viewers or cameras at night to take advantage of this fact. You may have seen cop shows or crime shows on television that use night-vision cameras to spot people or other living things in the dark. Warm bodies light up like a light bulb in this part of the spectrum.

The Science of Light and Matter

Spectroscopy is a branch of science that studies the interaction between light and matter. All elements have their own specific frequency of light to which they attuned, in a sense. These specific frequencies can tell investigators which elements or molecular compounds are found in samples that are either exposed to light or burned to radiate light.

Many elements were first identified on the sun through analysis of its spectrum, long before they were found on earth. Albert Einstein postulated, and proved, that light and matter were interchangeable, creating the equation $E=MC^2$. From this we know that light and matter affect each other in a measurable way, because they are different forms of the same thing. This might help to explain how light can affect the physiology of us humans.

How Color Therapy Works

In the practice of Color Therapy, shining the specific color of an element or vitamin may enhance the body's ability to assimilate and use it in the most effective manner. In this process, light may act like a catalyst that precipitates a process or event.

One of my own theories about this form of adjunctive healing therapy is that our bodies' cells may possess some mechanism that responds to light, perhaps in the same way that neuropeptides lock into receptor cells in our body. (See "How Our Mind Works" in Chapter 5 for more information on intercellular messages.) However, I do not know of any research presently investigating how light affects the body at the cellular level.

Many of us have known people troubled by seasonal affective disorder, or SAD, a condition caused by a general lack of light during the winter at certain latitudes north or south of the equator. We may have felt the "winter blues" ourselves, in certain regions of the country. Research shows that for the brain to release specific "feel-good" hormones into the body, it needs proper light levels. People living in far-north climes such as Finland and Iceland, or Canada and Alaska, where in winter months the sun is weak or disappears for months, sense a lack of light. They receive insufficient hormones, and then some experience the SAD condition. They can often be helped by sitting under a special lamp for some time each day. It's pretty simple. It is not strictly true that light as a concept is too exotic or intangible, too New Age, to consider as an important factor in our health.

Recently I saw a story on a nightly news program about a new product that made hair grow back in some balding folks or people with sparse hair growth. What was unique about it? It had zero side effects, and it consisted of a device (which resembles a hairbrush) that shines red light from LEDs (light-emitting diodes) directly onto the scalp, thus stimulating hair follicles to grow.

GOOD TO KNOW

A new study has found a direct link between **vitamin D** levels in the blood and lower incidences of cancer, including breast, lung, and colon types. The four-year study found that cancer rates for these types were reduced by about 60 percent when people took 1,000 international units (IU) of Vitamin D daily, an amount five times the current recommended daily amount (RDA) for people under 50.

Vitamin D is created in the skin when skin is exposed to sunlight. People who live north of the 37th Parallel might not absorb enough sunlight in the winter. In Color Therapy, violet creates vitamin D in the skin and can be used in the winter months when the sun lies too low. You can augment your vitamin D intake by increasing your time in the sun or by using Color Therapy.[8]

But set aside your thoughts about the ancients, and stained glass windows, and the winter blues. One reason that Color Therapy has been overlooked may be its *simplicity*. It consists of shining specific colors on your own body (or someone else's) by placing specialized gels or filters in front of a 90- or 100-watt halogen spotlight. An application requires one hour of colored light. The recipient then waits at least two hours before the next application. This means that, in a time of need, you can do eight applications of 1 hour each over a 24-hour period. The person being treated can be awake or asleep, reading or working. However, the light must be shone onto as much bare skin as possible in a reasonably dark room, with no direct sunlight coming in.

Treating Jaundice

When my daughter was born in 1982, she developed jaundice, in which the skin turns yellowish. Color Therapy uses the opposite color of a condition or illness to create balance; the opposite of yellow is violet.

Interestingly, hospitals have long used a type of light therapy to help treat jaundice, consisting of ultraviolet light that spills over into the violet part of the visible spectrum. In hospitals, staff cover the eyes of those babies being exposed to ultraviolet light, so as not to damage their eyesight.

I'm glad to report that after what amounted to my daughter's Color Therapy treatments shortly after birth, her jaundice disappeared completely in less than two days. I have known several other parents to have the same experience with their own babies.

Nil Side Effects

Happily, Color Therapy has no known side effects, although it interferes with proper digestion if done shortly after a meal. It is as if you were trying to digest two meals at once. Therefore, it is best to wait for two hours after eating before doing Color Therapy. The only color you can use immediately after eating is yellow, which will make what you have eaten more easily digestible.

Light Energy

You probably learned in your schooldays that everything we eat has captured or trapped light in it. This trapped light is somewhat like the electricity in a battery—it is energy stored there by chemical means. Plants use chlorophyll almost perfectly to absorb light energy from the sun, in order that they might create glucose and other compounds for their own needs. These compounds are molecules made up of hydrogen, oxygen, and carbon. Using the sun's energy, the plant takes up water (or H_2O) and carbon dioxide (CO_2) and then reassembles them to create new molecules, in the process that we know as photosynthesis. This synthesis of new chemical compounds is termed an *endergonic reaction*—that is, a chemical reaction in which more energy goes into the reaction than is released by it. The body's digestive system and other metabolic pathways are designed to free up this light energy by converting glucose and other compounds back into water and carbon dioxide.

As discussed in earlier chapters, our body breaks down the foods that we eat into their simplest compounds. It then liquifies them, to pass their nutrients into the bloodstream in the small intestine and stomach. In what is called an *exergonic reaction,* this breaking down of food releases some of the sun's trapped energy as light within the body. The pancreas regulates our metabolism by secreting insulin; this occurs when glucose in the bloodstream is absorbed and burned by the cells to release energy. This is called an *exothermic reaction,* which is felt as heat being radiated from the body.

Now, if you add up everything that goes into our body (through our mouth, skin, sinuses, or lungs) and then subtract everything that it eliminates (from our skin, lungs, sinuses, kidneys, or colon), what do you suppose is missing? The only thing missing is energy or light, provided that you maintain the same body weight. Of course, this light has not actually "gone missing," but it is the energy that was released by the chemical and metabolic processes of being alive. This demonstrates a universal law—that energy is never lost or gained in any chemical reaction. It is stored on one side of the reaction or released on the other side, or vice versa. Growing outside in the sun, plants absorb light energy, which we then take in when we consume plant and animal products, and finally we release that light energy. The matter changes only in chemical form, not in the amount.

Chlorophyll, mentioned earlier, is a molecule of green pigments that plants use in the process of photosynthesis, as they harness light radiating from the sun. Our own bodies contain a molecule that has a chemical makeup and structure almost identical to chlorophyll's—this is called *heme,* a component of hemo-globin found in our red blood cells.

Heme and chlorophyll are porphyrins, a type of molecule that binds with certain metals. The major difference between the two is that chlorophyll's central atom is magnesium, while heme's central atom is iron. This similarity is no coincidence, since all life on our planet shares a common thread—DNA. Some plants contain as much as half the same DNA as our own body. It may very well turn out to be a trait passed on from plants in our DNA that allows us to assimilate light, in a way that scientists do not yet fully understand.

At its most basic level, then, light is not a mysterious force of nature but rather an essential nutrient that we absorb through the skin instead of ingest, the way we take in food through the mouth.

TIP: LET THERE BE LIGHT

Light is a nutrient that is essential to most life forms, and certainly all humans. Light can be used therapeutically for many conditions.

Lemon Color to Detoxify

In Color Therapy, the color that causes the body to detoxify is often described as a shade of "lemon"—that is, a combination of green and yellow gels in a color lamp. If you showed this shade to people on the street, many of them would describe this color as "lime." These days new fire trucks are typically painted this color, as this is the frequency the eye is most sensitive to. This frequency, or color, is released by lemons when you eat them. If you eat no other foods than lemons, that color will dominate your body energetically and make your body detoxify.

Purple Color to Relieve Pain

When someone experiences a problem or feels pain while on the Master Cleanse, the cause can be toxins that have been stirred up and are moving out of the body faster than is comfortable for that person. In Color Therapy, purple slows cleansing and relieves pain, so to alleviate these symptoms you would shine purple on your body.

Purple is the opposite of lemon in Color Therapy, and therefore has an opposite effect. On Day 3 of my wife's first cleanse, she felt terrible pain in one knee, with some swelling. We were not surprised, for she had been diagnosed with rheumatoid arthritis of that knee. We immediately used a color lamp and shone purple on her, and I did some Vita-Flex as well. Not only did the pain go away, but she has never felt pain in her knees ever since—and that was more than 27 years ago.

Understanding the Primary Colors

One difficulty that Color Therapists must deal with is the lack of understanding about light and color in general. I have gone into bookstores and picked up as many as 12 books written specifically on Color Therapy, yet not one of them properly identified the three primary colors. That would be like a math book's not accurately explaining how to do simple addition or division.

When I give talks on this therapy, I like to test the audience by asking volunteers to name the three primary colors. Few people know the answer, unless they have read Stanley Burroughs's book, *Healing for the Age of Enlightenment*. When color televisions first came on the market in the 1960s, owners found it difficult to display proper skin tones, since the color dots used on the

---

What Color Is Your Aura?

I attended a workshop led by a woman who claimed to see light energy, which she called the human aura or the bioelectromagnetic field. When I signed in for the class, she told me at once that I had a temporary band of lemon in my aura, which she had also noticed with several others attending the workshop. At the time, I happened to be on the Master Cleanse. As it developed, the other people with the lemon aura were from my Vita-Flex class...and also were on the Master Cleanse!

TV screens at that time were red, yellow, and blue, which then were thought to be the primary colors.

Actually, the primary colors consist of red, green, and violet. This means that if you shine these three colors onto a white surface you will see only white light reflected back. To better understand this, take a prism and break up sunlight into the spectrum of its component colors; what you will see is red at one end of the spectrum and violet at the other end. These are the longest and the shortest frequencies of light that the human eye sees. Green is the other dominant color in between red and violet.

Below the color red in frequency is infrared. At the opposite end of the spectrum, the frequency above violet is ultraviolet. The color directly between the two is green. The primary colors create a balance; red is a hot color, violet a cool one, green a neutral one. Since green is neither hot nor cool, it has the properties of both. It can be used to stimulate rebalancing with all conditions. This makes up what is termed the *additive color system*.

People who paint (whether walls or pictures), who use dyes in their work, or who are in the printing business may tell you that the three primary colors are magenta (fuchsia, or purplish-red), yellow, and cyan (blue). This may be true for the specific use of colors whereby pigments, dyes, and inks are used to express color—known as the *subtractive color system*.

Practitioners of Color Therapy must understand the nature of light and how color is perceived through different expressions. White light is simply the blend of all colors, from red through the entire spectrum to violet. When you take a prism and allow sunlight to shine through it, the sunlight will be bent, or refracted, to create a color spectrum. This separation of the light into color happens because the different frequencies are refracted to their own unique part of the spectrum.

Now, when you take the three primary colors of magenta, yellow, and blue as paint, dye, or ink and mix them together in equal quantities, what do you get? Black. But why? When we view any object, what we actually see is not the object itself but rather the light reflected from it.

This is an important point to understand. The object we are seeing reflects back only a certain part of the spectrum. If the object is covered by paint, the light hitting the paint will be subtly altered. The chemical makeup of the paint makes it function like a light sponge. The paint interacts with the light by absorbing specific frequencies and reflecting others. The frequencies of light reflected determine what color you see. When you wish to paint a cabinet black, you can mix one paint that absorbs every color but magenta with another paint that absorbs every color but blue and a third paint that absorbs all colors except yellow. If you mix the three paints together in equal amounts, the net outcome is that all colors are absorbed and black is then created—black being the absence of light.

In Color Therapy, the three primary colors (red, green, and violet), when shone together, create white light. The three opposite colors (blue, magenta, and yellow), when mixed together as dyes or paints, create black. The first process works through light emanation or radiation, the second works by absorption and reflection of light. The sun and the moon are obvious examples of these phenomena.

GOOD TO KNOW

Primary colors = red, green, violet
Their opposite colors = blue, magenta, yellow
White = a blend of all colors
Black = the absence of light

White and Black

Black and white are not colors. White consists of all colors combined, while black is the absence of all light. Because light is an essential nutrient for the body and its good health, wearing black

---

Mellow Yellow

Several years ago I went camping with my daughter's seventh grade class. I was traveling in a car with a teacher and three students, going down a rugged logging road. We knew the trip would take about three hours on bumpy and winding roads. At some point, one of the young girls said she was getting carsick. I asked her to close her eyes and to imagine that she was completely surrounded by yellow light, as if she were inside a big yellow ball. After about five minutes of her sitting quietly and meditating on yellow, she suddenly said, "Why does that work?"

---

is best avoided at all times, except perhaps at funerals. Stanley said to avoid wearing black like the plague. (I'm not sure whether he meant the "black death," but he might have!)

When we wear black, the light that normally passes through your clothes to your body is completely blocked or absorbed by black. Many people who like to wear black are upset by what I say when I speak about color. Or maybe they are celebrities who are obsessed about their weight and looking "superstar thin" (since black clothes fool the eye somewhat). They just need to learn more about colors' effects on both health and mood.

Try Wearing Bright Colors

In my practice, when using Color Therapy on clients I often suggest that they wear brighter colors for at least two weeks straight, and then wear total black for at least a day or two. I ask them to be sensitive to how they feel different when donning black after two whole weeks of wearing colored clothes. I then advise them to assess their experience and go on to wear what feels best to *them*.

I myself prefer to wear many bright-colored clothes, and I am known for the way I dress.

The colors you wear and decorate your home with *do* have an effect on your life. Even imagining or visualizing color around your body can have an impact on your health.

Visualize Colors

It is likely that visualization of a color can have an effect similar to shining color directly on the body. This is another adjunctive therapy that can be used while on the Master Cleanse. Close your eyes, sit quietly, and visualize the following:

- Red, for vitality
- Orange, to help with constipation
- Yellow, for indigestion and low energy
- Green, for any other condition
- Blue, to help you relax
- Purple, for pain relief

This is merely a brief introduction to using color to optimize the results of your cleanse. You may wish to refer to Stanley Burroughs's book *Healing for the Age of Enlightenment*. In it you will find a complete discussion of Color Therapy, a description of the equipment required, color charts, and treatment programs to use when dealing with specific conditions.

The Resources section in the back of my book contains information about how to acquire a lamp and the gels needed to do color therapy.

CHAPTER 9

Essential Oils,
to Enhance Healing

Humans have used essential oils for many thousands of years. The ancient Egyptians incorporated them in many rituals, both as medicine and in the embalming process to carry the dead into the afterlife. When King Tut's tomb was discovered, for example, several clay jars were found that contained some 350 liters of essential oils that were still in a viable condition.

The Bible contains several references to essential oil. Many people know the story of the Three Wise Men who bore gifts of frankincense and myrrh (both precious incenses made from resin) to the baby Jesus.

The rediscovery of essential oils in the modern age happened, oddly enough, as the result of an explosion in a French chemist's laboratory in 1910. Working in his family's parfumerie, Dr. Rene-Maurice Gattefosse (who later coined the term *aromatherapy* and in 1928 published a book about it) was seriously burned in the accident. He thought quickly and applied the essential oil lavender, which happened to be on hand, to his burns. The healing process afterward was intense, but proved effective. The doctor called his healing substances "essential oils" (though they were not true oils), because they separated from water and looked like oil. The doctor shared this experience with Jean Valnet, a medical doctor in Paris.

Dr. Valnet began using essential oils during World War II—out of either necessity or desperation—when he noticed his supply of antibiotics dwindling. The beneficial results, as he tried various oils on wounds, led to him to share his newfound knowledge with two of his students, Dr. Paul Belaiche and Dr. Jean-Claude Lapraz. Both students went on to do clinical studies in which they investigated the myriad properties of essential oils.

In his books, Stanley Burroughs suggested the use of a few essential oils as simple remedies. Although he did not fully explore their potential, I hope to fuel your curiosity and desire to learn more about them. For me, essential oils have been the icing on the cake to Stanley's work—because they so immediately and effectively work together, synergistically. I do not travel anywhere without my kit of favorite oils, and when my children travel I always insist that they carry them as well.

What Are Essential Oils?

Essential oils are aromatic volatile liquids that have been extracted from various plants, flowers, trees, barks, and seeds by the process of steam distillation. These liquids are highly complex and consist of hundreds of organic compounds that, when blended together, create their unique smell. Essential oils are, however, much more than merely an aroma or scent. Their organic compounds, called constituents, determine their respective properties and qualities, which can sometimes have life-changing benefits on those who use them. Essential oils are made of plants' most potent parts. It often requires hundreds of pounds of fresh herbs to create a single pound of essential oil. Rose oil, for example, requires some 5,000 pounds of rose petals (if you can imagine that!) to extract just one pound of essential oil. It is this concentration-by-distillation that gives essential oils their power. The very term *essence* (which can be traced back to the Greek word for "to be") connotes something inherent in the plant, something derived from its basic nature.

An essential oil is not a true oil, unlike almond oil or olive oil, both of which are lipids. Essential oils are oil soluble—that is, they mix with oil. Essential oils float on water but will not mix with it unless they have been emulsified.

How Do Essential Oils Work?

Essential oils are composed of hundreds of constituents that make them *heterogenic* (meaning "completely different"). This is the crucial point to using them for health. Their many constituents possess numerous properties that work together synergistically, like a symphony orchestra whose many players are making music harmoniously as one unit. Oils' specific compounds, as well as their proportions to one another, determine the widely varied positive effects that people feel when using them. The manner in which they are applied to the body also affects how they work.

For example, when various antiviral drugs were first used in research trials to treat HIV-positive patients, initially they did not work very effectively. Then some scientists got the brilliant idea that they might work if mixed together as a "cocktail." And so it did; the "HIV cocktail" (in various formulations) now saves millions of lives each year around the globe. But nature already knows this! In nature, there are many essential oils that have proved to be extremely effective as antiviral compounds. Their effectiveness stems from the fact that they often contain hundreds of constituents, several of which are antiviral in nature—in other words, a cocktail of virus-fighting compounds.

By contrast, pharmaceutical drugs are often *homogenic*— meaning that only one chemical has been extracted from a plant or other source. This active ingredient is then synthesized and concentrated to make up the new drug. By design, this one compound now lacks all the other chemical compounds that, in its natural state in a plant or tree or flower or other element, were

> ## Saved by My Oils!
>
> In 2001, I was in Atlanta attending an essential oils workshop. During the proceedings, I suffered an outbreak of shingles, both the size of a 50-cent piece, one on my rib cage and another patch on my back. Those of you who have not had shingles should feel lucky. Shingles can feel itchy, irritated, and numb, and sometimes they even feel like an electric shock is being applied to your nerve endings. I knew that my condition was created by an acid condition in my body, which had allowed an opportunistic virus to come to the fore. At the emotional level, shingles can be caused by fear or worry.
>
> As soon as I could, I applied two different essential oils, without noticing any change at all. The two areas of shingles continued to itch and feel irritated until I got home, at which time I applied one drop of melissa oil (from the melissa plant, also known as lemon balm or bee balm; *melissa* is Greek for *honeybee*) on both areas twice in one day. By the end of that day both areas had completely stopped itching and the irritation and redness of the skin had vanished. Never since that time have I felt any discomfort in those areas. I have known people to have symptoms of shingles linger for several months without let-up. Melissa is a very powerful antiviral essential oil, plus it is calming and uplifting and helps to instill a positive outlook on life. Melissa now seems a logical choice for this condition, once you are familiar with its properties.

working in unison with it—with the goal of preventing side effects and creating greater positive healing activity.

Numerous clinical studies and books expound on researchers' knowledge of both heterogenic and homogenic drugs, with more results being published every year.

It turns out that essential oils are an important part of a plant's immune system, helping it prevent attack by yeasts, molds, fungi, viruses, bacteria, and even insects. Essential oils' complexity might, in fact, be an evolutionary strategy to keep these many different organisms from being able to adapt to just one chemical constituent. The plant, having been armed with several weapons, can launch an arsenal of attack against such invasive organisms and overwhelm them with hundreds of various chemicals.

Such a wide range of compounds lends itself to an extensive list of properties that each essential oil exhibits when used therapeutically. Among many other things, essential oils can do the following:

The Tansy Cure

I once heard a slim, older gentleman describe his experience with Idaho tansy and a chain saw. (I know that sounds weird, but read on.) The man had climbed into a tree to trim a branch, but after sawing through the branch he somehow pushed the roaring chain saw down across his lower leg. He quickly got down from the tree, and his wife put the essential oil Idaho tansy (which is related to the wormwood plant) on the wound. It stopped bleeding almost immediately. She used that oil because it was what she had in her pocket at the time. She drove him to the hospital, where doctors determined that he needed a bone graft and surgery. He refused and continued to use essential oils. As he was telling me the story, he pulled up his pant leg to show a scar about six inches long on the front of his shin. It had healed completely. I remember such stories, especially when I have seen the results with my own eyes or heard the incident described by the person involved.

- Thin the blood
- Stop external bleeding
- Reduce fevers
- Relieve pain
- Improve circulation
- Reduce acidity
- Reduce inflammation
- Act as an antispasmodic
- Help expel mucus from the body
- Act as an antimicrobial

Oils have another property whereby they become reactive to certain toxic chemicals in the body. This is often interpreted, wrongly, as an allergic reaction. Many of these same synthetic chemicals become stuck in the receptor sites of cells. Several constituents in essential oils will oxidize toxic chemicals and make for a healthy, functioning cell again.

Today about 300 essential oils are available on the market, online and in specialty health food and holistic stores. All are either distilled or extracted. All have a unique chemical makeup. All have a wide variety of properties and produce varying effects on the human body. Using a reference guide is vital for learning how essential oils work and knowing their proper application. But I have known of emergencies in which the only essential oil available was applied, regardless of whether it was the most suitable, yet good results were achieved.

How Are Essential Oils Applied?

There are three schools of thought regarding the most beneficial way to apply essential oils:

- Inhalation
- Direct application
- Ingestion

The first application, also called the German model, consists of inhaling essential oils from an air diffuser. This can create immediate changes in the brain, in both mood and function.

The most common and effective method for dispersing oils into the air is with a cold air diffuser. This device, which is readily available in a variety of models, blows air though the essential oil into a nebulizer, which creates a microfine mist that suspends oil particles in the air. The mist can float suspended for hours, clean-

---

Stops Bleeding Gums

A few years ago I needed to have a tooth extracted. The troublesome tooth had had a root canal procedure done years earlier. It is often thought that a dead tooth becomes a repository for many different microorganisms. When the dentist extracted the tooth, he put a piece of gauze over my bleeding gum and I drove home with it clenched in my jaw.

Soon after I got home my phone rang and I started talking in a muffled way, the gauze still in my mouth. I soon removed it and stayed on the phone for the next hour or two, talking to several clients about the Master Cleanse or other aspects of Stanley's work. But that constant talking kept my gum bleeding. Finally I told the person to whom I was speaking that I had to go fix a bleeding gum. I placed two drops of Idaho tansy on my gum where the tooth had been removed, and the bleeding stopped in less than one second. I continued to speak with people for another hour or so, and my gum never bled again.

Enhancing Mental Clarity

One day a woman called, wanting to purchase a color lamp. (See the Color Therapy chapter.) She was experiencing brain fog and fibromyalgia. I told her that I could deliver a lamp to her in person, so we set a time for the next day. She called later that same evening, to cancel her order. I asked her why she had changed her mind. She explained that her housekeeper felt she could not think clearly enough to operate such a device. I quickly responded by asking whether she could boil water. She said yes, of course she could. I then told her that she would be able to operate a color lamp and do Color Therapy.

The next day, when I delivered the lamp, I took with me a blend of essential oils high in sesquiterpenes. These are constituents of essential oils that research has found will pass through the blood-brain barrier and that therefore can affect brain chemistry. I placed the bottle under her nose and told her to breathe in the aroma, taking three or four deep breaths. I am sure that you have heard the expression "The lights are on, but no one is home." This woman was like that before inhaling the essential oil blend. Within a couple of moments, though, she was clearly present and alert and in control of her faculties. She quickly asked me about the essential oil and how it had worked.

---

ing the air as it kills both bacteria and many other microorganisms throughout the room. I like to use my diffuser when I host social events at my house, and many people comment on the wonderful smell.

To the uninitiated nose, therapeutic essential oils seem extremely strong upon first smelling them. A good way to start is to hold the bottle at waist level and let the scent rise up. Then slowly bring up the essential oil closer to the nose while continuing to sniff it. Some individuals may at first be overpowered by the strong aroma of pure essential oils, but become accepting of them as they familiarize themselves.

Most people are strongly attracted to oils when they are first exposed to them. There is another category of people: those who may not fully appreciate essential oils because of their exposure to perfumes, colognes, air fresheners, shampoo, and other products that contain synthetic fragrances. It may take some retraining of the nose, or a Master Cleanse or two, to reduce that sensitivity.

Direct Application

The second way to use essential oils is to apply them directly onto the skin, either neat or diluted with vegetable oil. It only takes one to three seconds to absorb an essential oil through the skin into the bloodstream, and usually at least 50 percent of the essential oil is absorbed. The half life of an essential oil is approximately 10 minutes, which means that if you absorb one drop into your body half is metabolized, or used, by the body in the first 10 minutes; in the next 10 minutes, it is again reduced by half; and so on, until it has all been metabolized after two hours or so. This rather quick absorption of essential oils prevents dependence or addiction, yet produces results that happen in mere moments but that can last indefinitely.

Two notes of caution: First, you must use therapeutic-grade essential oils. Second, your body must be alkaline, with a pH value of 7.0 or more. (See the "Water" section in Chapter 6 for a description of pH testing strips.) If your body is acidic, the oils can be reactive to the acidity in your body, which will create what some describe as an allergic reaction. If you suffer such a reaction, immediately apply a vegetable oil (such as cooking oil, olive oil, or canola) to remove the essential oils from the skin, and the irritation will quickly clear up. Soap and water will *not* remove essential oils from the skin but will only aggravate the irritation.

Combining Essential Oil Treatment with Vita-Flex

At this point you can probably appreciate my valid reasons for using essential oils in virtually *all* my treatments, especially during Vita-Flex. Experience has taught me that the use of essential oils is not limited by any modality or physical condition. I have met doctors, chiropractors, massage therapists, Trager practitioners, veterinarians, and myriad other practitioners who use and believe in their potential.

I have found that essential oils do not heal you, but instead they assist the body in re-creating balance or providing opportunities for healing to take place. I have also learned that essential oils do not always help people heal, unless they have a desire to heal. Let me explain with an example from my practice.

I was doing Vita-Flex on a female client. The big toe contains a reflex point that represents the jaw. When this point is found painful in Vita-Flex therapy, it most often indicates stress in the jaw caused by thoughts of anger or revenge. People touched on that sensitive point will often clench their jaw; some have even threatened to kick me.

When I asked the woman I was working on, "Who do you want to kill?" she smiled but refused to say, though she acknowl-

---

Treating Traveler's Troubles

I always travel with at least two small bags, each of which holds 16 small bottles of essential oils. Once, while flying to Hawaii, the plane encountered turbulence. The young woman seated next to me grabbed her air sickness bag to throw up. I quickly pulled out a blend of essential oils specifically made for digestive complaints, including nausea. I put four or five drops in her hand and told her to first smell it and then rub it on her bare stomach. Within a second or two she felt fine. The turbulence continued to escalate, to the point that I had to use the oil myself to forestall feelings of nausea. The pilot later told us that was the worst turbulence he had been in for years.

Years later, on another flight, I was walking back to my seat and saw lying in the aisle an obviously pregnant woman moaning, on her side. One flight attendant was bringing over an oxygen bottle and some ice, and soon another attendant helped her back to her seat. I offered my assistance, through the attendants. The pregnant woman said she would appreciate anything I could do that might help.

I went to my bag, took out the essential oil blend for nausea, and had her smell it, then asked how she felt. Only marginally better, she replied. I told her that I was surprised, because this blend usually helped nausea immediately. The woman responded that she was not feeling nauseated but dizzy! I said, "Sorry, but I brought the wrong oil," went back to my seat, and returned with another blend. I put about four drops on her right foot (the correct spot to treat dizziness). This appropriate oil worked and her dizziness completely cleared up. We went on to enjoy our flight home.

edged that it was true. I told her that she had to first express her anger and rage, and then forgive the person who had wronged her. She said she couldn't possibly forgive them. I replied, "You have to." And again she said she couldn't. To this I responded, "I will accept 'I won't,' but I will not accept 'I can't.'"

I continued to do the Vita-Flex, and when I reached the point where I rub the ears to stimulate circulation I took my chances and applied various oils to the client's ears. For this client I used a special oil blend that helps people forgive more easily. Scarcely three or four seconds passed before she said, "I think I can... What did you put on my ears?" She already knew what I had done, but had closed her mind to it.

This exemplifies how the oils sometimes work. It is as if they were opening doors that have been tightly closed for a long time in your mind. The door might open, but you still have to make the choice to step through the doorway and do the work that needs completion. On many occasions I have witnessed persons experienced with using essential oils helping to correct a number of conditions. I realize that their success was due largely to the fact that they were using therapeutic-grade essential oils, and they knew how to apply them properly.

Note, however, that essential oils can be reactive to synthetic compounds found in personal care products that have been applied to the body. What might appear to be an allergic rash may in fact be an interaction of the essential oils and these synthetic compounds that are in the fatty subdermal layers of the skin or in the blood. If you use a lot of personal care products, you might consider testing a small amount of essential oil on your skin. If you get an allergic reaction, immediately apply a vegetable oil to remove the essential oil. *Do not use soap and water.*

Ingestion

The third method for applying essential oils is to ingest them. They can come already encapsulated, or you can dilute them with vegetable oil or combine them with something like maple syrup to disguise the taste. I prefer to put my oils into empty vegetarian gel capsules, which can be purchased at health food stores. I use them almost exclusively while on the Master Cleanse, though they can be used anytime. The Food and Drug Administration has created a "generally regarded as safe" (GRAS) list for the consumption of essential oils.[9]

When taking essential oils internally, start with low dosages. Begin by using maybe one or two drops at a time. To err on the side of caution, you might consider dilution as a first choice.

I also use essential oils such as lemon, orange, peppermint, and grapefruit to flavor my drinking water. They are useful in cooking or baking because of their taste, but of course once heated they are no longer of therapeutic value.

While on the Master Cleanse I sometimes add one or two drops of lemon essential oil into each glass of my lemonade mix, to kind of supercharge it.

For people worried about having an overgrowth of *Candida* while on the Master Cleanse, one solution is to take essential oils during the cleanse. Clove, oregano, thyme, and cinnamon are effective choices, though all are caustic (hot to the skin) and should be used sparingly at first. You may want to dilute them, too. Do not consume more than what your body can comfortably manage.

I have heard some raw-food eaters express concern about using essential oils, since they are believed to be heated during processing. In fact, therapeutic-grade essential oils are distilled but not actually "cooked." The resulting product is stored in what are called cuticles—microscopic sacs that protect the oil from heat as steam liberates the oil from the plant. Once inside the condenser these cuticles, upon contact with cool water, burst open and free their contents. The oils then float in the water and are skimmed off into a collection tank. It is at this point that the constituents are sensitive to high temperatures.

Testing Oil for Purity

The most important information to someone who uses essential oils is whether they are of therapeutic grade. You do *not* want to use inferior-quality essential oils, for these can be contaminated, adulterated, or actually cooked.

An obvious question now comes to mind: If essential oils are so terrific, why would such a plethora of inferior oils be so readily available in the marketplace and online? The answers are two-fold: (1) greed and (2) ignorance. If I can produce a product that may sell for $10,000 a pound, I can double my profit by diluting the essential oil with a synthetic chemical that is not readily detectible by taste, color, or smell. Selling this inferior product to an ill-informed consumer becomes all too easy. I have warned people about the pitfalls of using inferior oils, yet some continue to purchase them because they are less initially expensive.

Inferior oils are made in a variety of ways. The plants can be grown using modern farming methods, including synthetic fertilizers, pesticides, and herbicides—all of which make for an inferior plant with petrochemical compounds that get into the distilled end product.

The distillation process itself can sometimes be suspect. While low-pressure and low-temperature distillation will not damage the oils' sensitive chemical structures, high-temperature and high-pressure processing saves the manufacturer both time and money but seriously compromises the quality of the essential oil being extracted. Oils damaged in this way can be further adulterated by the addition of chemical compounds (synthesized in labs) that are technically identical to those found in the plants themselves.

For instance, lavandin is a hybrid of lavender that produces considerably more essential oil than the true lavender plant (*Lavandula angustifolia*) but with a slightly different chemical composition. Lavandin contains a much higher percentage of camphor, so some unscrupulous manufacturers heat it to evaporate it, add synthetic linalyl acetate, and then sell it to unsuspecting consumers for half the cost of true lavender while promoting it as a good buy.

I always tell clients and colleagues that therapeutic-grade essential oils are well worth the price. (Would you want bargain-basement LASIK eye surgery, done in a dark alley?) I also tell them that if they don't see value in themselves, they will find it hard to pay for high-value things that they feel they truly deserve. Once again, money can be a determining reason why people will shy away from buying the highest quality or therapeutic-grade oils. I hope readers will thoroughly investigate the quality before they purchase any old essential oil.

Standards have been set by AFNOR (Association French Normalization Regulation) and ISO (International Standards Organization) certification, both of which determine, by a variety of laboratory tests, whether essential oils are of therapeutic grade by their chemical constituent profile. A gas chromatograph, which uses higher European standards instead of American ones, is used to measure the energy or light contained or held in the essential oil; this light quality determines whether the product is indeed therapeutic.

When essential oils are metabolized in the body, they release this same light that plants use from the sun to build their constituent properties. This, too, is a form of Color Therapy—essential oils are really liquid light! Each essential oil has its own unique symphony of colors or frequencies that will be released when applied to the body and metabolized in it. When purchasing essential oils, it is important that you ask your supplier to provide the results of GC (gas chromatography) tests made by independent laboratories specializing in the European standards set by AFNOR and ISO.

The details given in this chapter, and portions of the success stories that arise from my use of essential oils, may sound fantastic and implausible to some skeptical readers. But, just as I did, you may need to have your own experience with them to fully appreciate their wondrous healing power.

CHAPTER 10

Affirmations and Visualizations,
to Empower Yourself

The whole premise behind the Master Cleanse is *change*—that is, taking simple steps that give you a program for changing your experience of dis-ease to one of well-being. This opens the mind for a kind of brainwashing. As if the body were an older-model computer being refurbished, cleaned, and souped up with new memory and the latest nifty software applications, the process of cleansing the body physically helps make the mind more receptive to any new input, while deleting any unproductive programs that slow the system down or make it crash. This input is best implanted from a desire to reprogram yourself with an expected positive outcome.

Affirmations and visualizations are messages that you give, and repeat, to your unconscious mind—any number of beliefs and expectations that you specifically want to imprint on your unconscious. Some people find it simple and easy to memorize a few daily affirmations or to visualize certain desired end-states; for others, the process is a bit harder.

The mind works something like a computer, in that it can operate only with the instructions and beliefs that have been loaded into it ever since birth by interactions from your family, friends, community, and culture and that you modify by your own life experiences and what you tell yourself.

Computer programmers have a favorite saying: "Garbage in, garbage out." I use it here to suggest that, like a computer, the human mind can only function as well as its operating instructions and its full set of experiences and rules. If you have been programmed to constantly feel "ill," or to be "rejected" or "unloved," that will become your identity...until you change your internal program.

You Are NOT Your Illness

In my years of practice I have noted that many clients refer to themselves not as "I am Maria, with many wonderful possibilities lying ahead" or "I am Michael, and I deserve to be happy," but instead as their illness—"I am diabetic," "I am hypoglycemic," "I am always constipated," and so forth. People who do this are reinforcing their temporary or even chronic health condition, which usually leads to the belief that "Nothing ever works for me" or "I will never feel healthy again" and other self-fulfilling prophecies.

People use their illness as an excuse for why they cannot be successful, or find happiness, or say no to someone, or change some bad element in their lives. But be aware that using their illness as their identity can become a crutch that will be hard to throw by the wayside. To make the best decisions for ourselves, we need to feel empowered—yet if we never were empowered as children, it is hard to feel empowered as adults.

Most of what you know is learned early in childhood from your role models—typically your parents or guardians, or the people who raised you. I have many clients who, when they come in for a consultation, complain that have the bad luck to be "just like my parents," though as youths they swore to themselves that they would never ever be like them. This is the *nurture* part of our development, which affects us all as much as the *nature* part (our genetic makeup and inherited traits), or even more so.

Reprogramming Yourself

I will use another information technology analogy. To write a useful computer program, programmers must create or compile hundreds of thousands of lines containing flawless commands and instructions. If any one of the first three or four commands has an error, the entire program will need to be rewritten; errors elsewhere will cause the program to produce incorrect results, or even to stop running.

A child born in this world is similarly programmed and makes part of their reality such beliefs as "There is never enough," "I am not destined to succeed," "I am not good enough," and "Life is a struggle." Children today are inundated with these limiting beliefs—some actually verbalized by family or friends or teachers, some just absorbed subliminally through the culture. Can you see how a child who develops under this influence will shape their experiences in life to create or confirm distorted truths? In a way, we become psychological robots to fulfill the beliefs that we are given.

Fortunately, our consciousness is a more powerful force than the information that we were programmed with. We *can* change. While we cannot change the events of the past, we can change how we *feel* about them. To change, we have to let go of the old and the dysfunctional, in order to make way for the new and life-enhancing. The first step is often to recognize our limiting thought or belief, and the next step is to convince ourselves that we are willing and ready to release the thought and adopt a positive thought in its place.

In sessions with me, when certain clients become fixated on stressing their illness, or on self-identifying as their illness, I often suggest that they focus instead on our finding a path to well-being that we can sketch out together and then pursue. I urge them to

> ### Heart-to-Heart
>
> I was speaking with a woman in a health food store one day about a number of health-related topics, including the Master Cleanse. At least six times during this half-hour chat she said, "That just breaks my *heart!*" As I tried to wrap up the conversation so that I could get on my way home, she told me she was coming to my city for surgery. I said I was surprised that she had chosen to have surgery, because her attitude had not conveyed to me that she would be open to such an invasive process. I felt curious enough to ask, "By the way, what kind of surgery are you having?" She replied, "Open *heart* surgery—my mitral valve isn't working properly."

live in the present, prepare for the future, and not dwell on the past. Sadly, many times clients will interrupt me in five minutes or so, to tell me again how sick they really are. At that point I advise them to not speak of their illness again, or to just keep their mouth closed, until they get the point and can look at ways to make positive change.

Putting Your Mind to Work for You

Our mind will continue to go wherever we send it wandering. Would you rather run for *cancer,* or run for *life?* Too often, charities seem to be fixated on the very thing they are attempting to overcome. It seems like a no-brainer, but every year organizations ramp up a new war on something or other. Yes, it's good to help those charities that we wish to support. But do we want to constantly be in a struggle with our bodies, our health care givers, our insurance plans? Or would we rather be at peace with ourselves, with our bodies, with our minds?

To be fully empowered, we must accept responsibility for what we ourselves have created, rather than blaming ourselves or others (since we have all been exposed to similar types of conditioning). When we feel empowered, we can then take charge of our lives, and start living it as fully as possible. As we heal our lives, we inspire others to do the same. But we can only give away to others what we first give to ourselves.

On many occasions I have tested my clients by playfully asking them to give me a million dollars. They respond with variations of "I can't" or outraged cries of "Are you nuts?" I then ask, "Why can't you?" You can guess their reply: because they do not have such a sum. Love is like this, as well. You can't give love away unless you own it for yourself. Loving yourself then becomes the most important thing you can do for yourself. So stop all criticism of yourself and the others around you.

Finding the Secret to Big Dreaming

Some of you have heard about, or even read, a recent best-selling book that presents a certain "secret" to the world. The book has received a ton of attention in the media and on TV talk shows. But I never thought that the concept it conveys is truly a secret. Its ideas have been widely available for decades and are found in the writings of a number of American authors, dating back to the 1930s and '40s. These writings were largely ignored by the public until now. I have always assumed that many people just cannot or will not be responsible for the things they have attracted into their lives.

My own book and many other self-help books and therapies and practices all remind us that within ourselves we have the power to accomplish anything and that many people are truly open to new possibilities for growth, in a variety of life areas.

What has surprised me, though, is the backlash occurring to the teachings of that popular "secrets" book, which I view as being consistent with a most sacred American Dream. Most of us believe that, if you have a dream, you can make it happen in America. People come here from all over the world, immigrating legally or otherwise, because they know that here they can pursue their dream. Without dreams, there are no hopes, no expectations, no motivation. Dreams motivate people to work and strive for what they want. The "secrets" book does not advise you to sit on your behind and wait for the world to be served to you on a silver platter, but suggests instead that you work creatively and with intention so that the universe will respond in the way that you wish.

Fulfilling Your Dreams

I recently watched a program on the Apollo space program, and heard several astronauts discuss their lives, their space training, and finally their experiences of walking on the moon. One astronaut told of an incident from his childhood. He was outside in the garden with his mother, and when he looked up the moon was visible in the sky. He spoke to his mother and said, "Mom, someday I will walk on the moon." She, of course, replied that he was crazy and that was not possible. He should put that idea right out of his head, young man. He reiterated to her, "Yes, Mom, I will walk on the moon!" Sure enough, through hard work and focused commitment, he kept that dream—fulfilling it in his lifetime. So what is *your* personal equivalent of "walking on the moon"?

To put this into practice requires a lasting commitment. Start by listening carefully to the words you speak, and also to the thoughts and images that run constantly through your mind. Like a gardener, prepare the soil, plant good thoughts, water your garden well, then pick out and discard the weeds—and finally, take good care of the flowers and vegetables that please your eye and feed your soul and nourish your body. This all takes practice and commitment, of course, but with time it will become second nature to you and you will reap a healthy harvest.

Ideas for Affirmations and Visualizations

You can create reminders of affirmation-talk and positive visualizations in a variety of ways. Many books on the market—from religious to secular, from practical to philosophical—contain hundreds of soul-stirring affirmations that you can adapt to your own needs. The best ones are the ones that hit you in the heart; usually they are simple. People often have difficulty repeating or remembering a specific phrase. When that occurs, it is a signal that the affirmation hits home for that person.

Try a few of these affirmations, then add your own:

- I am becoming healthier day by day.
- The more I cleanse, the better I feel.
- I release the old to make way for the new.
- I deserve to be healthy, on all levels.

The simplest way to begin utilizing affirmations is to say them to yourself over and over, write them out repetitively at various times in the day, and post them in places around your home, your office, and even your car to remind yourself to think these new thoughts on a regular basis.

TIP

Some people are highly resistant to change. They might find it helpful to begin their campaign of positive self-talk with an affirmation that promotes change, such as this very simple one:
"I am willing to be well."

You might enjoy creating a "treasure map" or a "goals map" for yourself. Do this by making a collage of pictures and positive phrases cut from magazines, or found by browsing the Internet for quotations that really speak to you, or pulled up from your computer and printed. Such a map gives you a pleasant, vivid, visual reminder of some of your goals or intentions. Continue to refine them, of course. Post the map in a highly-trafficked place, like on a bedroom wall where you will see it both when falling asleep and when waking up, or in a prominent spot above the desk in your office, or on the fridge or over the kitchen sink.

Just visualizing or imagining whatever you like or want on a regular basis is also a highly effective tool for achieving your desires. You engage the imaginative part of your brain till you can feel it, taste it, hear it, and see it—until it becomes a part of your reality. It is important to remember that you *cannot* do this for someone else, nor they for you; they must create what they want from their own mind, and you must do the same.

Do a couple of these short visualizations, adding detail that makes them meaningful and memorable to you in your life situation:

- *See yourself about to step into a boiling-mad mud pot*, like you might see at Yellowstone National Park. With your first step into the hot mud you turn it into clear, blue, cool water and all the turbulence disappears! You rest yourself for ten whole minutes in the sweet calm of the water.
- *Visualize yourself in ideal health*. (For example, at your ideal weight.) See yourself living your life the way it would be if you had achieved your goal (say, being able to enjoy physical activities again, such as dancing or hiking or swimming). Visualize people in your life and hear them commenting on the positive changes you have made ("Wow, you look terrific!").
- *See yourself in a hallway with many closed doors*. Each doorway can be labeled with a part of your life that you wish to change (job, relationships, health, and so on). Choose a door to approach. Before you open the door, think: "I easily create the changes I desire." Now joyfully open the door and step through to the other side—where you will see the changes you want.

Above all, have fun with your affirmations and visualizations. Like eating a scrumptious ice cream cone, they should be a pleasure, not a chore. It can't hurt to think the best both *of* yourself and *for* yourself—even if at first you don't quite believe that doing so will have any power or effect.

This is only a brief discussion of the exciting topic of self-affirmations. Many books, CDs, and DVDs on the topic are available in bookstores and online. Please be good to yourself and read further on this subject.

CHAPTER 11

Parasite Cleansing,
to Reduce Your Toxic Load

Like toxemia, internal parasites are a problem of pandemic proportions. Also like toxemia, parasites are poorly recognized and little understood by most people. Parasites are organisms that range from single-cell structures to worms that can be as long as 40 feet. Parasites can be anything from yeasts and molds to fungi that infect the body and create dis-ease. Parasites are also directly related to toxemia, as they can only survive over the long term in a body that is unhealthy or toxic.

The problem with such organisms is that they live in your body at the expense of your well-being and good health. They are ill-mannered guests that will ruin your party! They not only live and go on to thrive in your body but, of course, they have to eat to survive—and this is where the problem starts. These microorganisms will dine on glucose, fats, and proteins from inside your body. They also have to eliminate—that's right, they dump their waste into your body. The waste they eliminate is toxic to it. These wastes, which are called mycotoxins, are extremely acidic.

Now, pardon me if I spoil your breakfast or your dinner along about now, but you should know that parasitologists have identified more than a *thousand* types of parasites that can survive in and inhabit the human body. That's your body and my body. Some scientists believe that there may be ten times that number, most of which have yet to be identified and therefore have not been treated with any precision at all.

Parasites' Nasty Behavior

Parasites, by definition, live off your body's cells. Many of them consume your blood for food. And as if that weren't enough, parasites such as intestinal worms can trap and hold waste in the colon, where they build "homes" or "nests" that protect them from attempts to rid your body of them. These homes are often misdiagnosed as tumors. I recently saw an image of the inside lining of someone's colon, with what looked like a tumor attached to the colon wall. The presenter said the object was, in fact, not a tumor but a parasite that had attached its home to the colon wall.

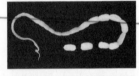

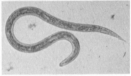

Top: The adult tapeworm of Dipylidium caninum *mainly infects dogs and cats, but occasionally is passed to humans by contaminated fleas.*

If you will excuse my indelicacy here, I have seen this very type of material eliminated while I was doing an advanced Master Cleanse! What is so interesting and weird about this is that I had been taking a number of herbs and essential oils to kill parasites for about two years prior to this advanced cleanse.

Bottom: Hookworm threadlike larva. Adult worms live in the lumen of the small intestine and attach to the intestinal wall, causing blood loss by the host.

Although the steps I had been taking probably killed many parasites, certain ones put up such a strong defense that it took extreme measures to get rid of them.

Some years back, while at a health conference, I met a man who claimed to have healed himself of liver cancer. He had been asked to speak at the conference about his journey to wellness. I was also presenting at this conference, on a different topic, and after we both finished our talks we spent several hours conversing on a variety of subjects. This man told me some details of his liver cancer and the various modalities that he used. As one of his interventions he had chosen surgery, but all the therapies that followed were alternative, by choice. At one point he told me that he had befriended several of his surgeons, so that he might gain a greater insight into his condition and what might be going on with his liver. His surgeons went on to inform him that many "tumors" that are thought to have attached themselves to people's livers are actually *parasites* coiled up inside that organ, and these are what doctors sometimes can successfully remove.

My Own Private Parasite

If you will allow me some personal revelations, I will tell you of my first experience with parasites, which began on the 33rd day in total of my doing the Master Cleanse in 1980. (Through the years I have kept notes as to unusual conditions or happenings during my cleanses, which is why I can mention this event here.) That particular day, after I had a bowel movement, as I was about to flush the toilet I noticed something unusual in it. It looked like a sausage skin, and was about three to four inches long. As I examined it more closely I realized it was no sausage skin at all (I didn't eat sausage) but was part of a parasite. I was quite freaked out to find that in the toilet, but was happy to have it coming out.

As I continued my Master Cleanse on and off throughout the year, I continued to eliminate what I was convinced were pieces of that parasite. This lasted for about 60 days of cleansing. One night while on the cleanse I woke up at about 4 o'clock in the morning to go to the bathroom, where I had a very unusual elimination in which I passed the head of the parasite. It had taken 90 days of noncontinuous cleansing to kill it completely and have it release and be eliminated.

Some of these sausage skin-like things that may appear in your toilet can, in fact, be linings of your small intestine or large intestine that are composed of mucus and who-knows-what-else. That "what-else" depends on your own diet and many other factors. Eliminating these unwanted visitors is a very good sign that this material is coming off, and that now your intestinal walls can start to heal and function optimally. You are on your way to better health!

Who on Earth Gets Parasites? (Almost Everybody)

In my first class on Stanley Burroughs's work in 1980, I was taught that probably 80 percent of the population were infested were parasites. I tell you, the class was not thrilled to hear that! A year or so later I heard a well-known herbalist lecture on parasites; he went Stanley one better and said that he believed that 95 *percent or more* of the population had parasites. He shared a few stories of his own experiences while treating people who harbored parasites. He told of a man who had come to see him because he could not keep any food down, but would throw up constantly.

The herbalist gave him a specific combination of herbs to stop his vomiting. Shortly after taking the herbal remedy he threw that up as well. The herbalist was now stumped, so decided to use a different strategy. The next combination of herbs that he used was one that deliberately causes people to become nauseated and to throw up. It did not take long until his client threw up two "nests" of parasites. I know that this does not make for pleasant reading, but it is extremely important that you understand the gravity of this problem.

About two years later I took another class on nutrition, parasites, and kinesiology. The instructor said unconditionally that 100 percent of the population had parasites, and that no one was

---

Bipolar, or Just Bugged?

Shortly after taking a class on parasites, I went to a party where I talked to a couple who seemed curious about the kind of work that I did. As I told them about my practice and specialties, the man seemed more interested, while the woman looked bored and didn't pay much attention to what I was saying. Then I mentioned how parasites can be related to bipolar disorder and other similar conditions. At that point the woman jumped into the conversation, and told me that her cousin, who had long been diagnosed as bipolar, had recently undergone surgery to remove parasites from her colon.

---

excluded. He recommended an herbal combination that was designed to kill parasites effectively. One day he spoke about a client he had been treating during his stay in our city. My instructor said that the evening before, a man called him up and asked him excitedly what he had done to the man's wife. My instructor replied, "I don't know. Who is your wife, and what *have* I done to her?" The man gave his wife's name, and said that she had "passed her bowels out of her rectum," or words to that effect. My instructor said that he had to see that, so he immediately hurried over to their home. When he got there, the woman was still sitting on the toilet—and two tapeworms were hanging from her rectum, one large and one small. Unpleasant but true story.

From that instructor, I went on to learn that the vast majority of illnesses or symptoms are associated with at least one or more parasites. He went on to say that many psychiatric conditions—including bipolar disorder, manic depression, and suicidal tendencies—are precipitated or otherwise affected by the waste that parasites dump into our bodies. which then poison the brain. This toxicity exacerbates any emotional state that we are experiencing, making us feel even more unbalanced and disassociated. The cure: Getting rid of the parasites, for starters.

Where Parasites Come From

Like viruses, yeast, bacteria, and other microorganisms, parasites are opportunistic. Just as certain orchids thrive only in the tropics on a mossy tree branch, parasites need a specific environment to live and grow in—that is, they need an unhealthy body. When a colon is overwhelmed with old fecal material, it creates an overacid condition throughout the body. Then whenever we are exposed to parasite eggs in our daily life, whatever the source, and we unwittingly ingest them, they have a perfect host in which to live.

Parasite eggs will float in the air that you breathe. They will sometimes be in the food you eat, or in the water you drink, or on the pets you love to touch. At least one type of parasite can burrow into your skin while you are in the water; I believe this is prevalent in Africa. People can also pass parasites to other people. There are many ways in which you can be exposed to parasite eggs.

Testing for Parasites

The gestation period of these eggs is extremely short—about 27 hours. This is important to know, because if you eat, digest, and then eliminate food in 20 to 22 hours or so, the eggs have no time to hatch in your body. This makes it critical that you find out the transit time of the typical food you eat. "Transit time" simply means the total time it takes from first swallowing food to the time it is eliminated from your body.

TIMED TEST FOR PARASITES

To figure this out accurately, swallow 2 tablespoons of sesame seeds without chewing them; use about 8 ounces of water (or one glass) to help swallow the seeds. Mark the time of day that you do this, and then start watching your bowel movements. When you see the first seeds in your stool, note that time, and continue to watch your eliminations to see how many eliminations are required to pass the seeds completely. If it takes more than 27 hours, it is very likely that you have parasites.

In addition to doing a timed test, there are physical indicators of parasites, such as an itchy nose or itchy rectum, or wavy fingernails, and of course bouts of constipation. The toxins that parasites release also tend to make people overemotional. Another accurate indicator on the mental and emotional level is when people feel too much like a victim, or feel that they are at the mercy of others or too much under their control.

One practitioner I know said that she found that the average person carries from 2 to 2½ pounds of parasites and their nests in their body. I cannot verify this, but I can say that our body, when healthy, may carry as much as 3 or 4 pounds of healthy intestinal flora. During advanced Master Cleanses that I have had clients do, I have seen many toilet bowls containing incredible numbers of parasites being eliminated, along with all the debris that they create and live in. People are first shocked when they see what comes out of their body during this intensive cleansing program. Then they usually become convinced that regular cleanses are a terrific idea!

How to Exterminate Your Parasites

I suggest to my clients and colleagues that they go out and buy an herbal parasite cleansing product, and use it while doing the Master Cleanse. You will always get better results when you starve the parasites while at the same time bombarding them with herbs that are toxic to their tiny bodies. Most antiparasitic remedies contain clove, black walnut, and wormwood, typically mixed with five or more additional herbs specific to each brand.

I also like to use essential oils internally, but repeat my caution that you *not* take any essential oils internally unless you absolutely know that they are of therapeutic grade (as specified in Chapter 9). I have learned that it's a good idea to rotate the various brands of antiparasitic remedies you are using, so as to hit the parasites hard with a variety of toxic elements. They may become somewhat immune to one particular remedy when exposed to it over and over.

It takes a considerable effort to get all the parasites out of your body. It will take extensive cleansing with the repeated use of antiparasitic supplements to achieve the desired results: a squeaky-clean colon free of yeasts, molds, fungi, and worms.

I like to do a parasite cleanse once or twice a year, to remain parasite-free.

See the Resources at the back of this book for additional information on parasites.

GOOD TO READ: ABOUT CLEANSERS

To find out more about parasites, browse the Web, using keywords like "herbal parasite cleanser." You may also wish to explore a variety of books on parasites, available at your local library or health food store or independent bookstore.

CHAPTER 12

Advanced Cleansing Techniques,
to Build on Your Successful Cleanse

I always feel excited when people come to me for ways to kick-start the cleansing process. In all likelihood that means they are both eager and committed to getting healthier. I too am continually looking for new and better ways to expand my repertoire of cleansing tools, both for myself and for my clients.

Many cleansing programs today require the assistance of a qualified practitioner. In fall 2005, for example, I experienced a 10-day cleanse using a colema board and consuming only a soft food diet. The diet eliminated all meat and dairy consumption and banned all wheat products. Foods with husks, peels, or seeds were also restricted under this diet. Before and during the cleanse, I took bentonite clay and psyllium husks twice a day.

Colema Board Cleansing

The colema board rests on your toilet, with one end on a chair or other support. You lie on it on your back; a hood covers an exit hole that empties into the toilet. From this hood comes a thin rectal tip that is inserted into your rectum about 2 inches. A water line is attached on top of the hood, which is then run to a 5-gallon bucket that contains purified water plus a combination of herbs. The herb mix can be varied, but most herbs used should be antiparasitic in nature. Each practitioner uses a different combination.

The bucket is typically hung from the shower head, using gravity to create water flow. An adjustable clamp is placed onto the water line so that the flow can be regulated or stopped by the person lying on the colema board. A colema cleanse is done once every day for 10 days, with 20 gallons of water used in each session.

The process lasts about 1½ hours per session and is similar to experiencing an enema. This process is not to be confused with a colonic, however. While both use water to flush or bathe the colon, that is where the similarity ends.

In the past I had felt hesitant to try such a process, but I had been pondering how to shorten the time needed to completely cleanse a colon of all its impacted wastes. A friend of mine chose to do the Master Cleanse, and decided to incorporate the use of a colema board. Her results were nothing short of amazing, which inspired me to try this process myself.

My experience with the colema board, and what I observed of other participants' experience, was revealing. Every day parasites were expelled, along with mucus, black ropey-looking things, and lengthy casings that appeared to be stripped from the colon wall. In one session, one person eliminated something that weighed about five pounds. Many people are astounded when they look into the toilet bowl and see what they have eliminated.

My first day of the colema cleanse in 2005 revealed a parasite in the bowel, which was a shocker—for I had been doing antiparasitic cleansing regularly for the previous two years. It turns out that in my cleanse I also began to eliminate the walls that parasites build to hide behind when you are trying to kill them.

Master Cleanse PLUS a Colema Board and Other Therapies

Just try to imagine how wonderful your own results could be, if you did the Master Cleanse in tandem with using a colema board, then added to it the following adjunctive therapies:

- A prolapsed colon lift
- Color Therapy treatments
- Some Vita-Flex sessions
- Perhaps even applications of essential oil

Depending on your condition and the time that has elapsed since your last cleanse, the Master Cleanse can require 40, 50, even 60 days or more in a row of cleansing to clear out *everything* from your colon. My own experience in 1980 was that it took about 90 days in total before I felt that my colon was quite clear. The parasite I finally succeeded in totally eliminating came out early in the morning on about the 90th day.

My point here is that 10 days on a colema board, when combined with all these adjunctive therapies, can do more for cleansing your colon than you could possibly accomplish with 50 days in a row of the Master Cleanse alone.

Whichever program you choose, there will be some trade-offs. The 50 days on the Master Cleanse will also do an extensive tissue cleanse throughout the body, and over the period of the cleanse will allow for a more effective healing of the entire digestive tract.

Understanding How the Colema Cleanse Produces Results

The colema cleanse is designed to directly address the waste stored in and parasites living in the colon. It gives a rather dramatic kick-start to cleansing. It's important to understand that the sooner you can cleanse your colon, the more quickly the Master Cleanse can get to the rest of the tissues in the body. These tissues have been poisoned by the continual onslaught from leaky gut or leaky bowel syndrome.

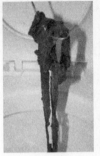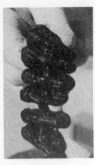

Left: Thickened mucus coating from the colon, which has become a host for putrefaction. Right: Rubbery encrusted fecal matter, result of a colon cleanse. Specimen's mucus lining took the shape of the bowel, complete with strictures.

This is all very workable in theory, but it requires determination and a commitment for all concerned (practitioner, patient, and patient's family). Cleansing can be quite difficult for many people, and some folks may not feel significantly better until six or even eight days into the schedule. Whatever the plan, people who choose to do a cleanse of any type need to be physically and emotionally ready for this demanding process.

Procedure for an Advanced Cleanse

The Master Cleanse is started the same day you begin using the colema board. There are a few changes to the regular program of the Master Cleanse, such as taking bentonite clay and psyllium husks for 5 days before starting the Master Cleanse. Combine 1 tablespoon of liquid bentonite and 1 heaping teaspoon of psyllium husk, mixed into 12 ounces of juice or water. Take this once a day for 2 days, and then twice a day for the next 3 days. You continue drinking the bentonite and psyllium husk mixture twice a day, mixed with the lemonade. You do *not* take the herbal laxative, however, because it is unnecessary while using the colema board.

GOOD TO TAKE: BENTONITE AND PSYLLIUM

Bentonite is a natural clay that comes from volcanic ash. Taken internally, it supports the intestinal system in eliminating toxins. The clay releases ions (sodium, potassium, and magnesium) in exchange for the substances they absorb. Bentonite clay comes in liquid form or in a powder.

Psyllium is a seed used for medicinal purposes. It is taken from the common fleawort plant, whose seeds and husks are harvested. Psyllium seeds are coated with mucilage that "bulks up" when exposed to water and stimulates the movement of material through the bowel. Psyllium is used for diarrhea and constipation and has been shown to lower serum cholesterol. Organic, without added sugar or color, is best.

For best results, use the colema board each day for the 10 days. This process will take about 2 hours each day.

When you finish using the colema board after a full 10 days, you can continue doing the Master Cleanse for as many days as you feel its benefits. The day you stop using the colema board you stop the use of the bentonite and psyllium husk mixture, and start using the herbal laxative teas twice daily. You come off the Master Cleanse by following the regular instructions in Chapter 6.

Refer to the Resources section for items and information mentioned in this section.

CAUTION

An advanced cleanse cannot be done easily without professional guidance. ***Do not try this on your own!*** If you are interested in pursuing an advanced cleanse, please be good to yourself and search out an experienced practitioner to guide you.

CHAPTER 13

Testimonials,
to Learn from Others' Experiences

Testimonial to the Master Cleanse

In 1998 I suffered a spider bite that brought on a huge reaction that raged through my body and its systems. It showed me how weak my immune system had become, and a slow thyroid function was detected. Over the next year some of the symptoms I had were random joint swelling and immobilization, kidney and liver dysfunction, strange rashes and purple mottled skin conditions and a persistent gray pallor, assorted back problems, digestive intolerances, colon issues, flus, fevers, colds and a persistent bronchitis that would not go away. The bronchitis I had had since childhood lasted usually the length of winter. In 1999 I ran into the Master Cleanse. After a year of trying every modality under the sun I was slightly improved but mostly maintaining a sorry condition.

Day 1 on the cleanse I had a cleansing reaction not 30 minutes after my first drink. Maybe I took too much cayenne but I broke out in a drenching sweat and was standing sort of helplessly in the middle of my bathroom wondering which end I was going to hug the toilet bowl with first, and forming a puddle on the floor. My metabolism shot up and I turned very red and was panting as well. About 20 minutes later it started to subside and I had impressive eliminations from many places but most impressive of all was a huge coughing fit in which I thought I had lost a whole lung—there was so much mucus.

Later that morning when I walked into my class everyone commented on how much better my pallor looked and I felt quite well. This started a series of cleanses for me and at last I started gaining some momentum in regaining my health. A year and a half later after 10 or 12 cleanses my conditions cleared almost entirely and I have had only one brief cold since, which is seven years ago this May. I also have not used any thyroid medications since that first cleanse.

—Tamara O.

372-Day Spiritual Cleanse

I met Tom Woloshyn at a essential oils training after which I scheduled him to come to my hometown to teach a 40-hour class of Stanley Burroughs's work, such as the Master Cleanse, Vita-Flex, and Color Therapy. I highly recommend that anyone going on the Master Cleanse take this course *in addition* to reading the book *Healing for the Age of Enlightenment*.

My first experience prior to that was a disaster. My "Iliad and Odyssey" has always been in pursuit of experiencing the ultimate, ultra, quintessential, optimum, degree of health—spiritually, mentally, emotionally, and physically ever after.

Having done colon, liver, and gallbladder cleanses as well as various water, fruit juice, and vegetable juice fasts of various lengths, I was the perfect candidate for the Master Cleanse. I had a suit of armor whose weft and warp were made from fibers labeled "fanatical," "extremist," "peculiar," "eccentric," "hard core," "black belt," "radical," "diehard," and my favorite, given by my then husband of 42 years—"stubborn." I was literally impervious to insult, criticism, and ridicule. It turned out to be a length of 372 days.

My original purpose was in quest of an answer I desperately wanted spiritually. But the plethora of rewards exceeded my imagination. Emotionally and spiritually I had never experienced the uniquely consistent and exorbitant high bliss, euphoria, and ecstasy. My weight maintained at 115 pounds in spite of the duration. I consistently jogged seven miles a day; no problem. I learned all the superfluous reasons people eat. Then I had a huge *fear* that if I was to resort to eating food, I would forfeit all my rewards of bliss, euphoria, and ecstasy. It turned out to be the most irreducibly minimal, simplest, effortless, experience pleasure for the most maximum results in my life.

—Maureen W.

My Master Cleanse Experience

I was out to dinner one night with Tom Woloshyn and some friends. I asked Tom about my doing a Master Cleanse, but I had concerns because I've had an allergy to citrus fruits since I was a little girl (I would get very bad hives, my throat would start to close up, and my entire body would become swollen). Tom assured me it would be OK as long as I did it exactly the way it's supposed to be done, with fresh juice, laxative tea, etc.

I decided to give it a try as my New Year's resolution and winded up doing the Master Cleanse for 12 days, making sure I only used organic lemons. It went without a hitch and I felt great (although admittedly quite nervous in the beginning).

The coolest thing is...I'm no longer allergic to citruses! I can very joyfully eat oranges, pineapple, and other citruses I've stayed away from, but greatly desired, since I was a child!

—Alice C., New Jersey

Cayenne and Citrus Allergy

I was wary of doing the Master Cleanse because I am allergic to cayenne pepper (hot spices generally) and sensitive to citrus fruits as well (though I honestly had only noticed reactions to oranges and grapefruit). Tom reassured me that he had seen people with such sensitivities do fine on the Master Cleanse and suggested I just go easy on the cayenne at first and see how it goes.

I took his suggestion and had no adverse reactions, even as I steadily upped the amount of cayenne I was using to the usual amount (1/10 teaspoon). There was no reaction to the lemonade either, and, being thin, I drank a lot of it. I did have some sensitivity to the orange juice in coming off of the Master Cleanse. I should have called Tom, as he later suggested that fresh mango or papaya (or pineapple as well, but I'm also sensitive to that) could have been used as a substitute.

—Ken S.

Tom's Workshop and Teaching

What Tom's workshop is, is an integration. Tom masterfully weaves this and that in his mix to create just the right ingredients necessary for understanding at a very deep level. It is not just a massage workshop like I thought it would be; it's an experience— A fits with B fits with J fits with X, and right back to A and B with a little D for good measure.

Tom is quirky, fun, and a great storyteller. Personal anecdotes are his preferred communication tool in the workshop I attended. Another, perhaps more accurate, way to describe Tom is that when you are in his presence, you learn just because of being there. He *is* what he teaches, and when you are open, you receive "it" automatically.

I am on the Master Cleanse now for 46 days. Looking back, I see the journey punctuated by "walls" that I ran into. What I found was that these perceived "walls" were in fact only in my mind, and stuck in my body (for me, specifically the digestive tract) in the form of emotions. So the Master Cleanse brought shifts on so many levels at various times. I almost quit at the first wall, which was Day 8. But I was at Tom's workshop when that happened and he made me aware of what was happening. Since then, I've moved through 5 or more "walls," and each time I did, more ease and beauty and Love awaited me; spiritual awakenings happening at such a seamless and rapid pace, one tumbling in after the other in perfect timing.

I'm not being trite. This has been the single most unique and expanding experience I have ever had (and I've had some amazing spiritual experiences). My journey of late has been masterfully enhanced and facilitated by Tom Woloshyn and his vast wealth of knowledge, teaching skills, and invaluable experiences.

If you have the desire to change your life, do the Master Cleanse now. If you have the opportunity to attend one of Tom's workshops, don't think—just do. Sign up immediately. I'm not saying it will be easy. It will be however you want it to be. But most certainly, it will be a journey you will remember very fondly.

—Zurino

Martial Artist Adds Eight Pounds of Muscle

I'm a 22-year-old, 4th-degree black belt Martial Artist who lives a very active lifestyle. I first heard about the Master Cleanse from my father. At the time, I was 18 and running 5K cross-country races, many of which I ran while on the Master Cleanse for 10 days at a time. Finding 10 days quite successful, I decided to cleanse a bit longer, so I did it for 28 days.

Throughout that time I watched my body, as lean (or "as skinny," I should say), change. My skin became brighter, the never-ending energy and strength I thought I had soared, and my thoughts and accuracy in and outside the Martial Arts just grew. And after weighing myself before, during, and after the 28 days, I found to my surprise that I'd gained 8 lbs of muscle. And to add 8 lbs to a then-142-lb. frame is nothing short of amazing....

I continue cleansing off and on until this day. I have also watched others cleansing, with some people losing weight and some gaining weight but all gaining health and strength in their lives. How could this be called anything other than the Master Cleanse!

—R. V. J., Georgia

Using Color Therapy

My biggest result from the light was when Martin and I went for a walk through a piece of land that was not level or even, but it looked safe to walk on. Little did I know that there were holes about 1 to 1½ feet deep, with grass covering them. Needless to say, I stepped right into one and went down hard. I didn't hit my knee, but stopped the fall with my arm. In trying to stop the fall I jammed my rotator cuff. The pain was so bad that I thought that I would pass out. I went home and the pain was getting worse every second.

I remembered the light, as I had just been to Tom's training on Vita-Flex and Light Therapy [Color Therapy]. I put green on first, to get the body ready to accept the light, and then I put on red for the pain. It seemed to ease some. I tried to lift my arm with such pain I could only lift it ¼ of the way up. I thought of the hospital, but I knew that pain pills would not help this!!! I waited about 2 hrs. and put the light on again. This time there was more relief, but it wasn't until the third time that I got a miracle. I put on the green light for the usual 20–30 min. and then I put on the red. This time I could really feel the light going in and pulling out the pain. My arm was released from the worst pain of my life.

I continued to use the light for the next two weeks and then I could lift my arm to a full range of motion. It really was miraculous.

My husband also had a wonderful experience. When I came home from the workshop with this "light thing" (as he called it), he was really mad. I told him of the science behind it and I thought that it may even help him. He had been in the house and in bed for about six months with extreme tiredness and no drive to do anything. He has been to many doctors, but to no avail. That night he went to bed and put on the green light and then changed to yellow. Within three days he was back working and did his biggest job to date.

Before this time we had already spent close to $200,000 in treatments, herbs and vitamins. So you can imagine that this was quite a surprise to us both. He still has his times, but it surely has been a great help to him.

—Kathryn Mc.

Maynard, Tom's Teacher

[The photos below are of Tom Woloshyn's teacher Maynard V. Dalderis. These photos were taken on July 31, 1978, and 60 days later on September 30. In the intervening time, Maynard studied with Stanley Burroughs, did 56 days of the Master Cleanse, and also used Vita-Flex. Maynard has for many years taught and promoted the work of Stanley Burroughs. He is the coauthor, with his wife, Leanne, of *Letting Go...One Step at a Time: Beyond Controloholism* as well as *The Gift Book* and three other Canadian bestsellers.]

What has set Tom Woloshyn apart from others as my most exceptional student is his willingness to put into practice these simple yet powerful techniques that yield results. Countless lives have been improved and actually saved by Tom's zest.

—Maynard V. Dalderis

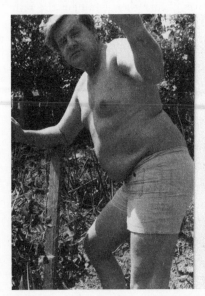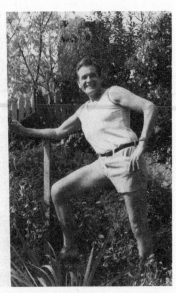

Maynard V. Dalderis before (left) and after (right) the Master Cleanse.

CHAPTER 14

Recipes,
to Improve Your Eating Style
After a Cleanse

I have included a few of my favorite personal recipes in this book. Over the years, many people who have done a Master Cleanse under my supervision have asked me to write and publish a recipe book, so that they would have a little boost after their cleanse when they are trying to adapt to eating better-quality food. Alas, I do not have enough recipes for such a project, but I thought I would contribute some of my favorites at the end of this book. Most are quite simple—and all are very tasty.

I am well known for my desserts. Although pies are my specialty, I did not include any pie recipes, but I did present a chocolate cake recipe. I derived this from a cake recipe that my aunt often used, but I have changed most of the ingredients to make it as healthy as possible.

Almost anyone can bake healthy things by substituting for poor traditional ingredients some of the natural and organic and vital products now available virtually everywhere and at any time of year.

I have a pet peeve. I travel a lot and shop in many health food stores, as you can tell by reading my many client stories in the previous chapters. I have noticed that the largest chains sell most of their baked goods with white sugar and white flour and any number of junky ingredients, as if they have no other choices. (What's up with that?)

Enjoy my recipes, and happy eating after your Master Cleanse! I encourage everyone to use as much organic food as is available to them. Many of the ingredients in the recipes that follow can now be found in regular grocery stores; otherwise, they can usually be found at health food stores. *Specialty items* such as chlorella, barley grass juice powder, or Bragg's Amino Acids are usually in stock at health food stores or can be purchased on the Internet. *Local and ethnic markets* can be a fine source for the freshest and tastiest ingredients.

GOOD TO USE: FRESHWATER ALGAE

Chlorella is a single-celled algae, used as a detoxifier, immune stimulator, and excellent source of general nutrition. Most forms of chlorella have been treated by cracking the outer cell wall, to aid in its digestibility. Chlorella is most commonly used to chelate, or remove heavy metals from the bloodstream. Take care to buy chlorella that is grown outside in natural light with clean water and no industrial pollutants. The Internet is a good source of information about this product. Health food stores carry it, in capsule or powder form.

Breakfast Smoothie

Fresh fruit

Fresh-squeezed juice

Fruit that you have previously frozen

Wolf berries or Goji berries

Barley grass juice powder

Chlorella powder

Water-soluble fiber (such as inulin or guar gum)

This is what I have for breakfast most of the time. In a blender I place fresh pineapple chunks, fresh papaya pieces, and fresh-squeezed orange juice and blend. To this I add a handful of frozen strawberries, raspberries, or blueberries that I had picked for myself in the summer and frozen.

I also add Goji berries (also called wolf berries) from the Ning Xia province of China. These berries are 16 percent protein and contain more vitamin C than do oranges, have more beta carotene than do carrots, and are very high in trace minerals.

I also add a little barley grass juice powder, chlorella powder, and a water-soluble fiber.

Blend well and drink.

To this smoothie, I often add various juices, such as cranberry, cherry, and pomegranate. In summertime when I have lots of fresh fruit on my kitchen counter, I like to vary the ingredients. One friend who lives in Southern California cuts up a well-washed lemon into her smoothie—peel and all.

GOOD TO EAT: GOJI BERRIES

Dozens of types of berries are called *Goji* berries, the best coming from China. These best-quality berries are super-high in antioxidants—almost off the charts issued by the U.S. Department of Agriculture, when compared to raspberries, Brussels sprouts, plums, broccoli, and so on. Goji berries offer many benefits, such as amino acids and polysaccharides. They are available online from several sources.

Coconut Almond Milk

¾ cup almonds

¾ cup shredded coconut (organic, unsweetened)

16 oz. of warm (not hot), water, plus more to fill the blender

1. Soak the almonds for 8 hours in water to remove the enzyme blocking agents. This allows the body to fully digest the almonds.

2. Place the soaked almonds in a blender and grind for 10 seconds.

3. Add the coconut and about 16 ounces of the warm water. Blend for ½ minute and then fill the blender up with warm water. Blend again at high speed for another minute.

4. Strain through a fine sieve or through cheesecloth, or through a cotton/poly blend of T-shirt material, into a pitcher. This recipe makes about 1 quart.

This milk tastes better than regular milk, is high in calcium and protein, and will keep for 5 to 7 days when stored, covered, in the refrigerator. It is also easy to digest. Use it to replace milk in all your recipes, and enjoy it instead of cow's milk when eating cereals.

If you use material to strain the mixture, either discard the material afterward or wash it well to release all the oils, otherwise they will go rancid in the cloth.

You can buy shredded coconut in bulk at most health food stores and some grocery stores.

Pea Soup

½ onion, chopped

1 10-ounce package of frozen organic green peas

Olive oil or coconut oil

3 cups coconut almond milk (see recipe above)

Salt to taste

1. Sauté ½ onion and the entire package of frozen green peas in a small amount of olive or coconut oil.

2. When cooked (about 5 to 8 minutes), put into a blender and add about 3 cups of coconut almond milk. Blend at high speed for 30 seconds, return the mixture to the sauté pan, and heat it to the desired temperature. Add salt to taste.

This is my favorite soup to serve to friends, because everyone absolutely loves the taste. The soup can be modified with any number of different precooked vegetables—try squash, broccoli, or cauliflower.

Mushroom Sauce

2 to 3 cups of mushrooms (several varieties, if available)

Onions, chopped

Garlic, minced (optional; use 1 clove for mild, or more if desired)

½ cup chopped celery

Coconut or olive oil

1½ cup coconut almond milk (see recipe earlier)

1½ tsp. tapioca flour

Salt to taste

1. Sauté the mushrooms with a small amount of oil (either coconut or olive). Add the onions, garlic, and celery.

2. When the mushrooms are finished cooking, add 1¼ cups of coconut almond milk. Reserve about 3 Tbsp. of the coconut almond milk and mix it with the tapioca flour, and then add it to the sauce.

3. Heat and let thicken. Add salt to taste and serve.

My family enjoys this sauce, which I like to serve over vegetables, or with whole grain noodles, or on wheat toast points.

Curry Sauce with Sautéed Vegetables

In this recipe you can use whatever vegetables are in season, or your favorites. Include some garlic and onions if you like them.

Vegetables of choice

Curry powder

Coconut oil

1 cup coconut almond milk (see recipe earlier)

1 tsp. tapioca flour

1. In a wok or steep-sided frying pan, sauté the vegetables until they are tender. Move the vegetables to the side. Place curry powder in the wok or pan, and add a bit of coconut oil. Heat the curry, stirring constantly for 10 to 20 seconds. In a small bowl, add tapioca flour to the coconut almond milk and pour into the wok or pan.

2. Cook the sauce for 2 or 3 minutes, and then mix in all the vegetables.

You can vary this sauce by adding 1 tsp. of tomato paste to the curry sauce.

Tom's Yummy Salad

1½ cups chopped cucumber

2 avocados, chopped

1½ cups chopped ripe tomato

½ cup extra-virgin olive oil

½ cup balsamic vinegar

Handful of fresh dill, chopped

Salt to taste

1. In a bowl, cut up the cucumber and lightly salt it.
2. Add the avocado and tomatoes to the cucumber pieces.
3. To make the dressing, combine olive oil and balsamic vinegar and mix well.
4. Add chopped dill.
5. Mix dressing lightly with the salad ingredients, and let sit for 5 to 10 minutes before serving.

This salad is always enjoyed in the summer, when its ingredients are at their finest. *Caution:* If you are sensitive to any plants in the nightshade family, you should omit the tomato in this recipe.

Quinoa Dish

1½ cups cooked quinoa

1½ cups frozen corn (or fresh, uncooked corn if available)

1 14-oz. can adzuki beans, or 1½ cups of your own cooked adzuki beans

3 to 4 Tbsp. hot salsa

Salt or Bragg Liquid Aminos

Monterey jack cheese (or cheese substitute), grated

2 sliced avocados (removed from skins and sliced into wedges)

1. Mix quinoa, corn, and beans together in a bowl. Add salsa to desired spiciness, and use either salt or Bragg Liquid Aminos to taste.

2. Put into a low baking dish, cover with grated cheese, and bake at 350°F. for 30 to 40 minutes.

3. Place avocado wedges on top of dish and serve.

Chocolate Cake

2 eggs, or egg replacer

2¼ cups whole wheat pastry flour

½ cup extra-virgin coconut oil

1 tsp. sea salt

⅞ cup raw cane sugar

¼ cup maple syrup

1 tsp. vanilla extract

½ tsp. baking powder

1 tsp. baking soda

⅔ cup cocoa powder

6 oz. coconut almond milk (see earlier recipe)

1 Tbsp. apple cider vinegar

¾ cup boiling water

1. Preheat oven to 350°F.

2. Mix cocoa powder and ¾ cup of the boiling water together, making sure that you remove all lumps.

3. In a large mixing bowl combine melted coconut oil, cane sugar, maple syrup, and then mix. Add 2 eggs and vanilla to the bowl and stir.

4. In another bowl, sift flour, salt, and baking powder together.

5. Mix 1 Tbsp. apple cider vinegar into the coconut almond milk.

6. In the large mixing bowl, add the cocoa and water mixture, the dry ingredients, and the milk with vinegar.

7. In a cup mix the baking soda with ¾ cup of the boiling water, then pour directly into the large mixing bowl. Mix all the ingredients together to remove lumps, but do not overmix.

8. Pour cake into a 9-by-12-inch pan (no extra shortening is needed) and bake at 350°F. for 50 to 60 minutes.

9. Check the cake with a toothpick to test whether it is done.

If the cake cracks on top when finished baking, the batter was too dry. Next time, reduce the flour by about ⅛ cup.

It is best to use "extra-virgin" coconut oil, as it has the best taste and is the highest quality.

For special occasions and parties, I am always asked to bring the dessert, such as my special chocolate cake, as above. The desserts I make are all natural and taste great.

Notes

1. On Dec. 10, 2006, *The New York Times* ran a feature story in its fashion section. The writer, Lola Ogunnaike, mentions "nutrition guru" Stanley Burroughs and some health-conscious people's vogue, in the 1970s, of purging their bodies of toxins. Recently a number of actors (Denzel Washington, Beyoncé Knowles) and models have done the cleanse to shed pounds before filming a movie role or doing a TV appearance; even a notorious New York City magician did the cleanse to toughen up his body. The article quotes several nutritionists who are less convinced of the cleanse's efficacy. Yet a *Court TV* anchor personality who did a cleanse reported feeling an "inexplicable burst of energy" by the fourth or fifth day.

2. Y. I. Goh, E. Bollano, T. Einarson, and G. Koren, "Prenatal Multivitamin Supplementation and the Rates of Pediatric Cancers: A Meta Analysis," *Clinical Pharmacology and Therapeutics* (2207) 81, 685–691, e-published Feb. 21, 2007. To contact the authors, visit gkoren@sickkids.ca.

3. Wyatt Webb, a psychotherapist and the leader and founder of Equine Experience at the Miraval Resort Spa in Tucson, Arizona, has written several books that deal with the topic of memories stored from childhood and their results on our lives. See his books *Five Steps to Overcoming Fear and Self-Doubt* and

What to Do When You Don't Know What to Do: Common Horse Sense.

4. J. H. Hankin and V. Rawlings, "Diet and Breast Cancer: A Review," *American Journal of Clinical Nutrition* (Nov. 1978) 31, 2005–2016. This article and many on the journal's website (www.ajcn.org) indicate that diet may inhibit or promote certain cancers, as well as other health conditions.

5. T. I. Ibiebele, J. C. van der Pols, M. C. Hughes, et al., "Dietary Pattern in Association with Squamous Cell Carcinoma of the Skin: A Prospective Study," *American Journal of Clinical Nutrition* (May 2007) 85, 1401–1408. To visit the journal's website, go to www.ajcn.org and search for keywords "skin cancer."

6. See Bernard Jensen, D.C., *Tissue Cleansing Through Bowel Management* (Escondido, Calif.: Bernard Jensen, D.C., 1980).

7. R. O. Young, Ph.D., and S. R. Young, *The pH Miracle: Balance Your Diet, Reclaim Your Health* (New York: Warner Books, 2003), 89.

8. J. M. Lappe, D. Travers-Gustafson, K. M. Davies, et al., "Vitamin D and Calcium Supplementation Reduces Cancer Risk: Results of a Randomized Trial," *American Journal of Clinical Nutrition* (June 2007) 85, 1586–1591.

9. Essential Science Publishing (comp.), *Essential Oils Desk Reference*, 3d ed. (Orem, Utah: Essential Science Publishing, 2004), 427. This book contains all the necessary information you need to use oils, instructions on using them correctly, lists of oils good for certain conditions, and contraindications.

Appendix

Resources

Stanley Burroughs Books

Stanley has two books or booklets in print: *Healing for the Age of Enlightenment,* and the *Master Cleanser with Special Needs and Problems.* These works can be purchased at health food stores or bookstores or online.

Tools

To purchase tools to maximize the Master Cleanse, such as color lamps, gels, and the Relax-a-Roller, contact Tom Woloshyn at www.vitagem.com; by mail at 3366 Cook Street, Victoria, B.C., Canada, V8X 1A8; or by phone at (250) 388-4102. The author's website contains a variety of information, including his speaking and workshop dates.

Visualizations and Affirmations

Louise Hay

Hay is the author of many informative and inspiring books. Her best-known work is *You Can Heal Your Life.* To listen to inspiring radio talks, go to www.hayhouseradio.com for a variety of positive programming.

Science and Positive Thinking

Many new books show the scientific basis and proof that *thought* is creative and can affect the physical world. Among them are the works of Bruce Lipton, Ph.D. (see his book in the Further Reading section). Lipton also has a website, www.brucelipton.com.

Essential Oils

Information

For information on how to obtain or use essential oils as an adjunctive therapy with the Master Cleanse, contact the author's website, www.vitagem.com.

Abundant Health

This source (www.abundanthealth4u.com) sells books and products related to essential oils, the labels mentioned on page 82 to charge water, pH strips, and a variety of Stanley Burroughs–related materials and tools.

Parasites

Hulda Clarke has created several protocols and devices for the elimination of parasites. For more information, visit her website, www.drclarke.net, or see one of her books, such as *The Cure for All Diseases* (India: Motilal Banarsidass, 2002).

A number of books now on the market deal with parasite treatments. See also *The Parasite Menace* by Sky Weintraub (Woodlands Publishing, 1998).

Advanced Cleansing

If you wish to do an advanced cleanse as described in Chapter 12, contact Tamara Olson at www.quantumleapcleansing.com.

Bernard Jensen

Dr. Bernard Jensen, D.C., was pivotal in promoting cleansing for many thousands of individuals throughout North America. Invaluable information can be found in his book *Tissue Cleansing Through Bowel Management*. Dr. Jensen's books, as well as supplies such as colema boards, can be obtained through his website, www.bernardjensen.org.

Food and Food Products

Bragg's Liquid Aminos are a Certified non-GMO liquid protein concentrate, derived from soybeans, that contains a number of essential and nonessential amino acids in naturally occurring amounts. The product is sold in many health food stores or can be purchased from the company, www.bragg.com/products/liquid aminos.html.

For Further Reading

Anderson, Richard, N.D., N.M.D. *Cleanse and Purify Thyself: (Book 1* and *Book 2) Secrets of Radiant Health and Vitality.* Mt. Shasta, Calif.: Christobe Publishing, 2000.

Burroughs, Stanley. *Healing for the Age of Enlightenment.* Reno, Nev.: Burroughs Books, 1976.

Emoto, Masaru. *The Hidden Messages in Water.* Hillsboro, Ore.: Beyond Words Publishing, 2004.

Essential Science Publishing (comp.). *Essential Oils Desk Reference* (3d ed.). Orem, Utah: Essential Science Publishing, 2004.

Finnegan, John. *The Facts about Fat.* Malibu, Calif.: Elysian Arts, 1992.

Foundation for Inner Peace. *A Course in Miracles.* Mill Valley, Calif.: Foundation for Inner Peace, 1975.

Gray, Robert. *The Colon Health Handbook: New Health Rejuvenation* (10th ed.). Reno, Nev.: Emerald Publishing, 1980.

Hawkins, David R., M.D., Ph.D. *Power vs. Force: The Hidden Determinants of Human Behavior.* Carlsbad, Calif.: Hay House, 2002.

Hay, Louise, L. *Heal Your Body*. Carson, Calif.: Hay House, 1982.

———. *You Can Heal Your Life*. Carson, Calif.: Hay House, 1984.

Hendrix, Harville, Ph.D. *Getting the Love You Want: A Guide for Couples*. New York: Harper Perennial, 1988.

Higley, Connie, and Alan Higley. *Reference Guide for Essential Oils*. Spanish Fork, Utah: Abundant Health, 2006.

Jensen, Bernard, D.C., N.D., Ph.D., *Tissue Cleansing Through Bowel Management* (Escondido, Calif: Bernard Jensen, D.C., 1980).

Lipton, Bruce, Ph.D., *The Biology of Belief: Unleashing the Power of Consciousness, Matter, and Miracles*. Mountain of Love (publisher), 2005.

Pert, Candace B., Ph.D. *Molecules of Emotion*. New York: Scribner, 1997.

Svoboda, Katerina, and Tomas G. Svoboda. *Secretory Structures of Aromatic and Medicinal Plants: A Review and Atlas of Micrographs*. Middle Travelly, Beguildy, Knighton, Powys, U.K.: Microscopix Publications, 2000.

Vanderhaeghe, Lorna R. *The Body Sense Natural Diet*. Mississauga, Ont., Canada: John Wiley & Sons Canada, 2004.

Vasey, Christopher, N.D. *The Miracle Grape Cure and Other Cleansing Diets*. Rochester, Vt.: Healing Arts Press, 2006.

Williamson, Marianne. *The Gift of Change: Spiritual Guidance for Living Your Best Life*. San Francisco: HarperSanFrancisco, 2004.

Young, Robert, O., Ph.D., and Shelley Redford Young. *The pH Miracle: Balance Your Diet, Reclaim Your Health*. New York: Warner Books, 2003.

Cleansing Journal

START date: _____   **END date:** _____

Weight: _____   Weight: _____

Measurements: *Measurements:*

Chest: _____ Waist: _____   Chest: _____ Waist: _____

Hips: _____ Thighs: _____   Hips: _____ Thighs: _____

Energy level on a scale of 1–10   Energy level on a scale of 1–10

(1 = lowest): _____   (1 = lowest): _____

Start your cleanse the night before with an herbal laxative.

	In a.m., herb laxative *or* 32 oz. water w/2 tsp. noniodized sea salt	Number of 10-oz. lemonade drinks (6–12)	In p.m., herb laxative	Number of bowel movements	Notes
sample	7:30 a.m. tea	╫╫ |||	8 p.m. tea	9:15 a.m. 9:30 p.m.	A bit tired
Day 1					
Day 2					
Day 3					
Day 4					
Day 5					
Day 6					
Day 7					
Day 8					
Day 9					
Day 10					

Notes on Your Cleansing Journal

Keeping a journal while doing a cleanse will help motivate you, by showing each day's progress. If you run into a snag, refer to previous days' entries on the chart or reread the appropriate section of this book to come up with a solution. If you plan to do more than a single cleanse, keep all your journals to document your success over time.

Tip: Photocopy this spread and make your entries on it.

Important: Before you start the Master Cleanse, *please read this entire book* and make notes or highlight passages that seem to apply to your situation. Then you will know how to cleanse correctly, how to come off your cleanse, and know what to expect along the way.

But first, complete the following statements.

I am doing the Master Cleanse because:

_____

_____

Before starting the Master Cleanse, I am feeling:

_____

_____

Have someone shoot a few photos of you, pre- and post-cleanse, to remind you of how you looked and felt. If you are keeping a separate journal book too, complete the above statements in the book; paste in your "before" and "after" photos, and any "goal photos" you spot in a magazines; and write down your favorite affirmations (see pages 152–54).

In **column 1,** record when you take your morning herb laxative (whether tea, tablet, or capsule), steep time or dosage, and any discomfort such as cramping; adjust dosage as needed. —OR— Write down when you drink a *salt water bath*, its measure, and any deviation from the usual salt-to-water ratio (page 68).

In **column 2,** mark each day's lemonade drinks that you consume. Be sure to drink at least 6, but no more than 12. Record if you add more than 4 Tbsp. of maple syrup and the amount of cayenne (page 69). Hydrating yourself well helps you detoxify.

In **column 3,** log in the time you take the evening's herb laxative.

In **column 4,** mark the times of each bowel movement, plus any helpful details (type, consistency, color).

In **column 5,** write how you feel each day, physically and emotionally. Write down your wins and detox symptoms—anything you are learning about your body and how it responds to a cleanse. If you wish, track sleeping patterns or energy levels here, also.

Index

Other Ulysses Press Books

Complete Colon Cleanse: The At-Home Detox Program to Restore Good Health, Boost Vitality, and Ensure Longevity
Edward Group, $12.95
Packed with info on powerful, all-natural cleanses as well as advice on long-term colon health, this book is the ultimate tool for relieving colon-related illnesses, restoring vitality, and obtaining maximum colon health.

Do-It-Yourself Guide to Biodiesel: Your Alternative Fuel Solution for Saving Money, Reducing Oil Dependency, and Helping the Planet
Guy Purcella, $15.95
Contains the most current and complete information available for making biodiesel at home.

The Easy GL Diet Handbook: Lose Weight with the Revolutionary Glycemic Load Program
Dr. Fedon Alexander Lindberg, $10.00
Using these more accurate and sensible GL scores, *The Easy GL Diet Handbook* offers a plan for healthy weight loss and reduced risk of diabetes that's easier to follow. It also includes numerous foods that the Atkins, South Beach, and GI diets wrongly consider "off-limits."

The GL Cookbook and Diet Plan: A Glycemic Load Weight-Loss Program with Over 150 Delicious Recipes
Nigel Denby, $12.95
Offers a vast selection of GL-scored recipes so dieters can choose dishes they love while following a proven program for permanent weight loss without hunger.

Irritable Bowel Syndrome: A Natural Approach
Third Edition, Rosemary Nicol   foreword by William John Snape, $14.95
Clearly written with easy-to-understand explanations, this book presents natural solutions for living comfortably with this common ailment.

The Juice Fasting Bible: Discover the Power of an All-Juice Diet to Restore Good Health, Lose Weight and Increase Vitality

Sandra Cabot, $12.95

Offering a series of quick and easy juice fasts, this book provides a reader-friendly approach to an increasingly popular, alternative health practice.

The Liver and Gallbladder Miracle Cleanse: An All-Natural, At-Home Flush to Purify and Rejuvenate Your Body

Andreas Moritz, $14.95

Illustrates how to recognize stone buildup and provides do-it-yourself instructions for painlessly flushing them out of the body.

Mastering Cortisol: Stop Your Body's Stress Hormone from Making You Fat around the Middle

Marilyn Glenville, $15.95

Details specific ways to counter cortisol with a tailor-made exercise plan that will slim the belly. Based on breakthrough genetic tests, the program also recommends specific vitamins and minerals and explains which foods will work best for the reader.

The pH Balance Diet: Restore Your Acid-Alkaline Levels to Eliminate Toxins and Lose Weight

Bharti Vyas & Suzanne Le Quesne, $12.95

Tells how to pH-test one's body, correct imbalances, and eliminate toxic overload by following a dietary way of life that works. An easy-to-follow section with over 40 recipes is included to help guide readers through the plan.

To order these books call 800-377-2542 or 510-601-8301, fax 510-601-8307, e-mail ulysses@ulyssespress.com, or write to Ulysses Press, P.O. Box 3440, Berkeley, CA 94703. All retail orders are shipped free of charge. California residents must include sales tax. Allow two to three weeks for delivery.

About the Author

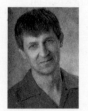 Tom Woloshyn began practicing and counseling in holistic health methods in 1980, after taking a course in the healing techniques of Stanley Burroughs. His main focus of expertise includes the following modalities: the Master Cleanse, Color Therapy, colon lifts, Vita-Flex massage, the mind–body connection, detoxification, and the use of essential oils. He maintains a holistic health practice in Victoria, British Columbia, Canada.

Over the last 25 years Woloshyn has expanded his knowledge by working with a variety of teachers, including Burroughs himself, as well as by treating thousands of individuals. To share what he has learned, he has lectured and led workshops all around the world. He has also produced a DVD program, titled "Vita-Flex: The Instructional Video with Tom Woloshyn," that demonstrates the correct use of the technique.

He is deeply committed to providing individuals the opportunity to better understand the body and the healing process, and to improve their own health and lives. He believes that, when people are given enough information, they will choose the proper path to wellness.

Tom Woloshyn welcomes inquiries and feedback. He can be contacted via his website, www.vitagem.com, or by telephone at (250) 388-4102 (please call after 9 a.m., Pacific time).